MOOD FOODS

MOOD FOODS

William Vayda

Ulysses Press Berkeley, CA

1995

Published by: Ulysses Press
    P.O. Box 3440
    Berkeley, CA 94703-3440

Library of Congress Catalog Card Number: 94-61103

ISBN: 1-56975-023-8

First published as *Psycho Nutrition* by Lothian Publishing, Australia

Printed in the USA by the George Banta Company

10 9 8 7 6 5 4 3 2

Editor: Beverly Zegarski
Cover Design: Design Works
Cover Illustration: "New Woman" Diane Ong/Superstock
Editorial and production staff: Jennifer Wilkoff, Lee Micheaux,
    Doug Lloyd, Mark Rosen
Indexer: Sayre Van Young
Color separation: Pro Scan

Distributed in the United States by Publishers Group West and in Canada by Raincoast Books.

Printed on recycled paper

Acknowledgments

My graditude goes to three of the most brilliant minds in psychiatry. The true pioneers, Dr. Richard Mackarness, Dr. Abraham Hoffer, and Dr. Bernard Rimland, who have inspired and informed me. From them I learned the twin principles of nutritional psychiatry and clinical ecology. I would also like to thank the many Australian scientists and doctors who have contributed to and helped with my knowledge and experience.

CONTENTS

INTRODUCTION

Psychonutrition is the popular name given to the branch of medicine that deals with nutrition and its effect on the mind. This branch of medicine, orthomolecular psychiatry, looks at the effects of natural chemicals, such as vitamins, minerals, and amino acids, on the brain's chemistry.

In the 1950s, two psychiatrists, Dr. Abraham Hoffer and his colleague Dr. Osmond, discovered that certain people showed signs of mental illness if they were deficient in vitamin B_3 (niacin) and that other people's mental illnesses could be helped by administering large amounts of certain nutrients that were either deficient in their diet or for which these individuals had unusually high requirements. Both groups using nutritional therapy improved considerably, and many individuals completely recovered.

Even though the niacin treatment was successful and a great deal less harmful than the standard psychiatric regimen of the 1950s (electroconvulsive therapy [ECT], insulin shock, and psychoactive drugs), the orthodox scientific community was, and still is, slow to acknowledge these findings. Many great scientists, including the late Nobel Prize winner Linus Pauling (who in 1968 wrote a memorable article titled "Orthomolecular Psychiatry" for *Science*), were looking for more links between nutrition and mental illness. Within a few years a host of vitamins and several minerals were found to help the niacin treatment, and so orthomolecular psychiatry became a complex therapy involving a formidable array of nutrients.

At the same time, other workers in the field discovered that fluctuations in blood sugar (hypoglycemia), which could occur independently of vitamin deficiencies, were also capable of causing a number of physical and mental disorders that mimicked many psychiatric

conditions. Many patients regained their health as a result of understanding that diet, as well as vitamins and minerals, could influence
mental health.

Dr. Richard Mackarness, a psychiatrist at Basingstoke District Hospital
in England, had studied and applied the findings of Dr. Theodore
Randolph, a leader in the study of allergies, to mentally ill patients.
After much success with nutritional therapy, Dr. Mackarness wrote a
book called *Not All in the Mind*, which was first published in England
in 1976. For the first time the average person, as well as professionals
in the field of psychiatry, could read a simple, yet shattering, account
of diagnostic and treatment methods that were brilliant in both their
simplicity and their effectiveness.

Psychiatry and our understanding of human behavior and brain biochemistry took a giant leap forward: we learned that while vitamin
and mineral deficiencies, or dependencies, still played a major role in
orthomolecular psychiatry, it was pointless running blood tests for
vitamin deficiencies or glucose tolerance tests for hypoglycemics
when we could first find out if they were hypersensitive (allergic or
intolerant) to some foods, certain chemicals, or even airborne environmental factors. Any of these hypersensitivities could be "causing"
nutritional imbalances and deficiencies by promoting malabsorption;
they could equally "cause" hypoglycemia by placing such a stress on
the body's ability to cope that blood-sugar levels would plummet
anyway!

Later, we discovered that an overgrowth of *Candida albicans* (candidiasis) could also cause, or be caused by, any or all of the above factors,
and so it became more and more obvious that we had to start by
eliminating the major factor at hand rather than the underlying
cause. For example, if hypoglycemia were causing someone to be
stressed and this manifested as an allergy that allowed candida organisms to grow unchecked, we would have to start treating the over-
growing bugs (or the presenting symptoms). Once they were taken
care of, then the allergies and blood-sugar problems would be dealt
with. If the problems did not improve, then we would look for any
independent causes.

Perhaps as a legacy from orthodox medicine, some people still have
difficulty accepting that it is quite possible for a psychiatric patient to

suffer brain-chemistry dysfunction caused by a deficiency of niacin while also being hypoglycemic because of diet—without the two being necessarily related in a cause-and-effect continuum. While correcting the hypoglycemia with diet changes will make the patient healthier, the psychiatric problem will not be taken care of until supplementary niacin is given. Conversely, treating the vitamin problem and the hypoglycemia as well as the food allergies or intolerances may not ensure good health while the patient is exposed to airborne molds or dust.

The latest and most promising nutritional treatment, known as *precursor therapy*, is now routinely employed by all of us in treating candidiasis and yeast-related problems. Precursor therapy makes use of pure amino acids that are the precursors of most, if not all, of the brain chemicals or neurotransmitters that control our moods. For example, a patient with allergies or an infection, such as candidiasis, may also suffer from depression. In such a case, the administration of an amino acid, such as DL-phenylalanine or perhaps L-tyrosine, will reduce depression while the treatment for the other condition is carried out. This is possible because both amino acids are precursors of brain chemicals that act naturally as antidepressants.

It is the ability to keep an open mind that has characterized many of the great scientists, and it is my hope that this book not only informs a great many readers but also encourages all of us, including the orthodox medical community, to keep an open mind and to look for better, more simple, and less harmful ways to help our fellow humans.

MEMORY: HOW TO IMPROVE IT AND THINK CLEARLY

CHAPTER 1

If you wish to maximize your brain functions, including memory, it is a good idea to start by learning something about how the brain works.

How the Brain Works

The human brain is an irregular globe of moist, jelly-like tissue containing more than ten billion nerve cells called *neurons*. Each neuron has numerous root-like fibers with tiny bulbs at the ends. Minute amounts of chemicals known as *neurotransmitters* burst out of these bulbs continually and hit the walls of other brain cells. Once these other cells are charged, they fire their own neurotransmitters, and this activity is repeated millions of times each minute of our lives.

Learning, memory, moods, sleep, appetite, and sex drive are all controlled by neurotransmitters. In fact, we literally cannot make a move without them, because they also control the coordination of our muscles.

We also have controllers of these controls: more chemicals. We are not sure what they all are, but we do know that diet influences the type and amount of neurotransmitters. Vitamins and minerals are involved, in fact essential, in the production of these brain chemicals from ordinary amino acids extracted from the proteins in our daily food.

There are some 30 known neurotransmitters and probably many more that we don't yet know about, all of them made from amino acids. Food is broken down into individual amino acids, which then enter brain cells and are converted to neurotransmitters in a series of biochemical steps that cannot take place without the presence of several essential vitamins and minerals. That is why it is possible to treat emotional and psychiatric problems with highly individualized diets and nutrients, such as vitamins and amino acids.

If someone is allergic, is hypersensitive, or has an intolerance to some foods or the chemicals that they contain, these can cause the brain to react adversely and therefore cause a sort of "brain-allergy" reaction. Placing such patients on a diet that avoids these sensitizing foods or chemicals can often cure or greatly help their condition. However, in many cases, simply changing a diet so that it includes the appropriate amino acids for the required neurotransmitters does not work satisfactorily. That is why we usually prescribe amino acids as supplements, which is known as precursor therapy.

Dietary manipulations do not work satisfactorily because most foods contain a number of amino acids that all compete to get to the brain.

Precursors

Precursors are the substances, in this case a dietary or supplemental amino acid, from which the brain makes a neurotransmitter. Following is a short list of some of the amino acids and the main neurotransmitters that are derived from them.

Source/precursor	Neurotransmitter
choline/serine	acetylcholine
glutamic acid	glutamine/gamma aminobutyric acid (GABA)
histidine	histamine
lysine	citrulline, pipecolic acid
phenylalanine	tyrosine, dopamine, norepinephrine
tryptophan	serotonin
tyrosine	epinephrine, norepinephrine

As there are only a limited number of "seats" on the blood-to-brain bus (see "The blood-brain barrier," later), too many amino acids of one kind will stop others from even getting on the bus.

For example, turkey contains lots of tryptophan (an amino acid the brain turns into serotonin), which makes people sleep well. Many similar foods contain an excess of "competing" amino acids, and eating them will give little benefit if eaten at bedtime in order to treat insomnia. If, however, you take some carbohydrates (say, a tablespoon of honey) at the same time, this will help elevate blood sugar and inevitably cause the release of insulin. Doing this has the unusual effect of chasing several amino acids from the blood into the liver. However, insulin does not have this effect on tryptophan, which now that all the other competing amino acids have been shunted to the liver, has the brain bus all to itself, and there is a good chance you will get a good night's sleep.

As you can see, it is not enough to know what to eat. You must also know when to eat and how to combine your food if you want to influence brain chemistry via diet. This, of course, is something we all do on a daily basis without ever realizing it.

The answer is not simply taking amino acids as supplements, because they will not always work and can sometimes make matters worse. The key is to take only those supplements that are needed for particular individuals depending on their circumstances. This applies to almost every diet, pill, or potion, but especially so to anything that may act on the brain.

We are all biochemically unique, and what may put one person to sleep may keep another awake all night. For instance, tryptophan can act as a stimulant for a heavy drinker.

THE BLOOD-BRAIN BARRIER

As cells go, neurons are particularly frail. Their functions can be disrupted by an incredibly large number of toxic substances and "natural" molecules, such as amino acids, that are normally present in the blood but kept away from the brain's private circulation.

For example, folic acid, a nutrient regarded as a vitamin, is essential for the body's good health. Normally very little folic acid is allowed to pass from the bloodstream into the brain's circulation. However, when too much folic acid does enter the brain, it can cause convulsions. In fact, a group of drugs used for the treatment of epilepsy act precisely as *antifolates*. Antifolates are substances that antagonize folic acid (which is also known as "folate.")

A complex barrier has evolved in the human brain to keep it isolated from general circulation. This selective filtration system, known as the *blood-brain barrier*, normally allows only oxygen, glucose, and a few selected nutrients to penetrate it. While the knowledge of how the blood-brain barrier works is invaluable in designing drugs that will act on specific neuron complexes, it is equally important in deciding which nutrient may play a role in altering brain functions.

Psychobiologists have discovered that the behavioral effects of many drugs, neurotoxins, and "foreign" molecules occur precisely because of their ability to disrupt, or modify, the orderly chemical transmission between neurons. We also know that "mental illnesses" may be caused by excessive, insufficient, imbalanced, or defective neurotransmitters. And practically all these neurotransmitters are made from common components of the foods we eat every day.

NUTRIENTS FOR THE BRAIN

Despite its relatively small size, the human brain consumes more energy than any other organ. Representing only 2 percent of total body weight, the brain uses 20 percent of the total resting oxygen of the body.

Most people know that the brain cannot function without oxygen and that brain damage follows after even a small period of time without. However, what must be understood is the underlying reason why oxygen is crucial to brain function. Oxygen is needed to make glucose, the primary source of all brain energy. If the flow of oxygenated blood to the brain is interrupted, an individual will lose consciousness within ten seconds. A little longer without brain oxygen may cause permanent brain damage. It is also worthwhile to note that similar effects can be caused by any condition that lowers blood-sugar levels (these are discussed under "Hypoglycemia" on page 34).

Cuddles and Brain Power

Intelligence, brain power, memory, and just about every activity the brain performs are greatly dependent on the formation of new connections. In addition, the protein content of each cell is constantly being destroyed and remade.

This building activity is largely dependent on the stimulation of nerve fibers, which occurs whenever our central nervous system is busy.

Even just touching, stroking, or cuddling a child can have an enormous impact on its future intelligence potential. Babies deprived of physical contact have fewer neuron connections and may become mentally and physically stunted.

There is, in fact, a well-documented syndrome called *deprivation dwarfism*, caused by a lack of sensory inputs to an infant. "If you don't use it, you'll lose it" is an old adage that applies as much to brain power as to libido, memory, and muscular strength.

Therefore, a prerequisite for optimal brain power is a good supply of oxygen, which is transported to the brain by the blood. Good blood flow is critical if we are to use our brain efficiently.

There are many ways to improve your circulation: regular exercise and special yoga positions; a good massage given by expert hands; chiropractic manipulations, which free previously restricted blood supply to the brain by correcting spinal and neck dislocations; and acupuncture. In addition to physical methods of increasing circulation, there are several nutrients that play a role, such as vitamin E, vitamin B_3 (niacin), and ginseng.

Because blood-sugar supplies are so critical to brain functions, you should ensure that glucose levels in the brain do not fall too far or too rapidly. A condition known as *hypoglycemia* (low blood sugar) can play havoc with anyone trying to think clearly. Two of the most common causes of hypoglycemia are unsuspected food allergies or intolerances and *candidiasis* (systemic thrush). Another syndrome that often appears simultaneously with low blood-sugar levels, and may either be its cause or one of its effects, is hypoadrenocorticism, which occurs when adrenal glands are exhausted.

Nutrition plays a central role in the treatment of all these conditions, so chemicals that the brain uses to make its own special foods and that are readily available in your diet are a good place to start looking for ways to improve your brain function. Follow a well-balanced diet with a reasonable amount of proteins, some complex carbohydrates, no refined sugars or sweets, and small, frequent snacks, rather than few large meals.

The Two Memory Banks

It has been proposed that memory is stored in two different parts of the brain: a short-term memory bank, where events are recorded for a relatively short period of time, and a long-term memory bank, where events are transferred from the first bank. Unless information is transferred from the short-term to the long-term memory bank within a specified period, it is lost forever.

In the late 1940s, Donald Hebb, a psychologist at McGill University in Montreal, proposed that when neurons receive repeated stimulation from nerve cells they become more and more sensitive to the signals. As a result, information becomes encoded in the more permanent memory. We all know that repeating information, such as saying a telephone number more than once, makes us more likely to remember it. Today we still do not know how the brain remembers, let alone where the memories are stored, but Hebb's theories remain the best explanation we have.

There are several factors that can interfere with memory. Several commonly used drugs are known to adversely affect memory. Lorazepam, a tranquilizer, can be used to help people forget unhappy experiences. Some digitalis-like drugs used in the treatment of heart disease interfere with the electrical impulses to the brain that are necessary for memory storage. They may also inhibit the synthesis of proteins, which is thought to be used for encoding memory.

It would seem that any drug that affects the central nervous system, whether a tranquilizer, narcotic, sedative, analgesic, or antipsychotic, has the potential to adversely influence human memory.

The Hippocampus

By 1973 Tim Bliss, of the National Institute for Medical Research in London, and Terje Lomo, of the Institute of Neurophysiology at the University of Oslo in Norway, had narrowed their research on memory to a part of the brain known as the *hippocampus*. This small structure is believed to be essential for memory.

We know that even animals that are quite low on the evolutionary scale can learn. The hippocampus appears to be an important element for learning. Scientists have demonstrated that repeated electrical stimulation of hippocampal neurons over long periods of time makes brain cells more sensitive to stimulation.

The brains of people suffering from alcohol-induced damage can often be found to have impaired hippocampal functions. According to several orthomolecular scientists, zinc deficiencies can render the hippocampus inefficient.

Whether taking zinc supplements can increase memory remains to be seen. However, we already know that zinc, which reduces the level of copper in the brain and in turn excites brain cells, can produce a degree of mental relaxation, reduce lead accumulation, and improve the conditions of some schizophrenics and alcoholics.

Serotonin and Tryptophan

Serotonin is associated with sleep, moods, and perception. Too little serotonin may cause sleeplessness, depression, and difficulties with temperature regulation. Too much serotonin may be involved with premature aging, psychosis, sleeplessness, and aggressive behavior. Although no direct connection between serotonin and memory has been found so far, it is interesting to note that people who find it difficult to fall asleep tend to be deficient in, and helped by increased levels of, this chemical. Sleeping pills, while helpful, do not promote deep, restful, rapid-eye-movement (REM) sleep.

According to Dr. James McConnell, professor of psychology at the University of Michigan, REM sleep, which is associated with dreaming, may well be the key to long-term memory storage. "Dreaming," he says, "may be what happens as the new memory molecules go out of where they have been stored during the day. This triggers old memories, which is what we experience as dreams. That is why dreams appear to relate to what happened during the day. Other findings indicate that if you prevent REM during sleep, you have no memory."

The synthesis of serotonin requires considerable amounts of vitamin B_6 (pyridoxine). It is interesting to note that a deficiency of this vitamin can be associated with lack of dreams because serotonin increases the REM portions of our sleep. (For a list of foods high in vitamin B_6, see page 11.)

The brain makes serotonin from a common amino acid called tryptophan, which can only enter the brain by a mechanism known as active transport. Tryptophan shares this mode of entry, however, with several other amino acids, and so taking tryptophan may not increase

Foods Containing Tryptophan

alfalfa	egg
baked beans	endive
beef	fennel
beets	fish
broccoli	milk
Brussels sprouts	nuts
carrot	soybeans
cauliflower	spinach
celery	sweet potato
chicken	turkey
chive	turnip
cottage cheese	watercress

brain serotonin levels unless the number of competing amino acids is also kept low.

Two ways of enhancing tryptophan's transport across the blood-brain barrier are by fasting (tryptophan should always be taken well away from mealtimes) and by eating carbohydrates, which tend to cause the pancreas to secrete insulin. Insulin in turn depletes the blood-stream of precisely those amino acids that are competing with trypto-phan for transport across the blood-brain barrier.

While manipulating tryptophan and serotonin levels can be helpful in various conditions, it would seem that memory is worsened, if anything, by increasing tryptophan dietary intake (*New Scientist*, Oct. 1983, p. 47). This probably happens because the increased brain levels of serotonin, which follow the intake of tryptophan, make the brain cells more sleepy.

While increased brain levels of serotonin may help some people to sleep, too much may make them unable to rest and become aggres-sive and suffer hallucinations.

Memory Rhymes

Exercises to improve memory, known as *mnemonics*, have been known for thousands of years. The ancient Chinese used to make rhyming poems of long lists of names in order to help them remember.

Psychobiologists believe that the brain can mark up only seven separate items, or "chunks," of information on the blackboard of short-term memory at any time. The items more likely to be shift-ed to our permanent memory bank are those that create vivid visual images or strike a connection with something particularly eventful in our lives.

This is what mnemonic exercises are all about: a way of making otherwise boring information into something that has meaning and is interesting. A string of letters such as GTR will be remem-bered much more easily if we associate it with the word *alligator* and make a visual image of it.

Excessive levels of serotonin have also been associated with premature aging and fetal damage. A deficiency of serotonin can cause depression, sleeplessness, and even psychiatric disorders.

Fast Thinking: Glutamic Acid

Fast thinking and memory go hand in hand and require speedy communication between brain cells. The major signaler in the human brain appears to be a simple amino acid called *glutamic acid*.

Glutamic acid acts in practically every brain cell to cause rapid excitation, and, in fact, it seems to be the most common "on" signal used by sensory nerves entering the brain. This fact alone would make glutamic acid the most important neurotransmitter for encoding information, that is, memory. And it may well be one of the reasons why so many researchers claim that glutamic acid appears to "clear" the head and enhance such functions as thinking and remembering.

Glycine, another amino acid, is known to be an inhibitory transmitter at the spinal cord, but the best-known inhibition effect in the brain may well be that exerted by gamma-aminobutyric acid (GABA). Having a fast car with a responsive accelerator won't get you far if you are unable to slow down when you need to, so inhibitory neurotransmitters play a central role in brain functions and at least a powerful, if indirect, one in memory. Roughly a third of all nerve cells in the brain send inhibitory rather than accelerating signals, and the chemical they use (GABA) is closely related to glutamic acid. In fact, these two are among the most common amino acids within the brain and spinal cord.

VITAMIN B$_6$: TOO MUCH VERSUS TOO LITTLE

GABA is manufactured exclusively in the brain and spinal cord from glutamic acid and is particularly reliant on ample supplies of vitamin B$_6$ (pyridoxine).

Glutamic acid, from which the brain makes GABA, excites, while GABA inhibits. When vitamin B is deficient, glutamic acid can reach excessive levels, perhaps causing irritability of the central nervous system. Additional intake of vitamin B$_6$ could increase the sedating effects of GABA both by allowing more of it to be synthesized and by reducing accumulated glutamic acid. At the same time, an excess of vitamin B_6 may deplete glutamic acid reserves to the point where proper excitation and hence perceptive functions of the nervous system are impaired.

This relationship may also account for the observed correlation between dreaming and vitamin B_6 status. This correlation is one of the commonly used diagnostic methods for a naturopathic assessment of vitamin B_6 levels in patients. Its role in memory function is peripheral at best, but being unable to relax mentally could influence one's ability to memorize facts during a heavy period of studying for exams, for example.

Glutamic acid, like most amino acids, does not easily cross the blood-brain barrier, so eating more foods rich in glutamic acid, or even taking glutamic acid as a supplement, will have little effect. Fortunately,

Foods High in Vitamin B_6 (Pyridoxine)

avocado	meat (beef, ham, pork)
barley	milk
beans	molasses
Brazil nuts	oranges
carrots	peanuts
cheese	peas
cow's milk	potato
crab	prunes
egg	rice
fish (cod, halibut, herring,	soybeans
mackerel, salmon,	spinach
sardines, tuna)	sunflower seeds
lentils	wheat bran
lima beans	whole-meal flour
liver (pork)	yeast (brewer's)

the brain can make its own glutamic acid from substances normally found in the diet. If the diet is low in these substances, then impaired brain function may occur.

Glutamic acid can be used by the brain as fuel if and when blood-sugar levels are too low. It can also pick up and remove excessive ammonia, which tends to build up during brain activity. In addition, ammonia is associated with aging, so its prompt removal may help to keep brain cells younger and, therefore, smarter.

Glutamic acid has at least two other important functions. It helps to reduce the craving for alcohol, and it plays an important role in maintaining the efficiency of the immune system.

The only practical way to increase brain function with glutamic acid is by taking it in the form of L-glutamine, which is a compound that can cross to the brain and be converted to glutamic acid as required. L-glutamine has been reported to increase the IQ of patients with low IQs.

A CASE OF POOR MENTAL FUNCTIONS AND MEMORY

Peter is a lawyer who complained that his work efficiency had decreased dramatically in the past few months.

"I don't seem to be able to concentrate as well as I used to, and my memory simply disappears when I most need it," Peter moaned. "At first I attributed it to stress, overwork, that sort of thing. I took a holiday and had a good rest. Naturally, I felt a lot better, but my brain still refused to get into gear."

I asked Peter if he experienced his difficulties all day long or only at particular times of the day.

"In the morning, when I get to work, I am not the best, and by lunchtime I can't think straight. I feel a little better after lunch, but by 4 p.m. my concentration is all but gone."

I explained to Peter that the most likely reason for his problem was that at certain times his blood-sugar levels might fall too low. This condition is called hypoglycemia, and it works in the following way. Some of the food we eat is converted into blood sugar. If the food contains a lot of sugar or consists of refined carbohydrates, like pastry or white bread, this tends to flood the blood with sugar too quickly. The body responds to this by sending out signals that cause hormones, such as insulin, to pour out in an effort to decrease the high blood-sugar level. The faster and more massive the blood-sugar elevation, the greater the insulin response. Then the blood-sugar levels drop quickly and deeply, stopping the brain from functioning efficiently. This reaction can be prevented by eliminating sugar and refined carbohydrates from the diet and by eating small and frequent snacks. There are also supplements that can be taken to enhance brain power.

I prescribed L-glutamine, phenylalanine, tyrosine, ginkgo, vitamin B_{12}, and vitamin B_6: all nutrition factors that are involved in the formation of neurotransmitters, the "chemicals to think by."

I also recommended to Peter that he try several different types of breakfast and lunch foods to see which enhanced his mental powers. I explained to him that some of us are fast oxidizers and others are slow oxidizers. In other words, some people burn carbohydrates quickly, while others burn them slowly. Therefore, it is not uncommon to find some people who function well on a breakfast of eggs, butter, and whole wheat bread but cannot get any energy, mental or otherwise, from breakfast cereals. At the same time, many individuals find that if they eat anything but carbohydrates in the morning, they feel lethargic and tired. They do well on breakfast cereals, skim milk, a little jam on their toast, and a cup of coffee.

Peter took my advice and, to his surprise, found that if he ate a boiled egg for breakfast and took his supplements, his brain would take off in top gear as soon as he began work. When he switched back to carbohydrates, the old symptoms would come back within a few days, although less severely because of the supplements. In addition, the tyrosine increased his ability to cope with stress, and he found that phenylalanine reduced his craving for sweets.

Peter learned a very important lesson in nutrition: we are all biochemically different, and, while general recommendations, such as eating less fat, less sugar, and more fiber, can be beneficial to most people, we should always try to find what is best for each of us rather than following generalizations.

Memory and Acetylcholine

Acetylcholine is a chemical substance secreted at the ends of many nerve fibers that is responsible for transmitting nerve impulses. Acetylcholine levels in the brain are said to correlate with memory functions. Certain conditions which produce memory loss, such as Alzheimer's disease, are associated with decreased levels of acetylcholine. Additionally, we know that drugs that block the action of acetylcholine in the brain cause a temporary loss of memory function.

Unfortunately, supplementing choline, the amino acid the brain uses to make acetylcholine and to help improve memory, has failed to produce consistent results. However, this may be due to the fact that vitamin B_5 (pantothenic acid) and vitamin B_1 (thiamine) are needed to convert and use choline as acetylcholine. Perhaps if these nutrients were administered in the correct amounts, together with lecithin or choline, memory enhancement would occur.

Another way to increase brain levels of acetylcholine, and a method that has been shown to be effective in promoting good memory, is a prescription drug called Dianol (dimethylaminoethanol-p-acetamido-benzoate), only available in the United States by special order from European sources. It has been used successfully in treating memory impairment among the aged and in hyperactive children. Dianol can also be useful in the treatment of depression, apathy, and senility.

In addition to increasing acetylcholine levels, Dianol helps the body to get rid of lipofucin, which are aging pigments that show up as dark spots on the skin of older people and can also be found in the brains of people suffering from senility.

Dr. Richard Hochschild, an American gerontologist, has also found that Dianol can increase the lifespan of laboratory animals. Unfortunately, Dianol is a drug and may therefore have unknown side effects. There is, however, a natural compound called *deanol*, introduced by Dr. Carl Pfeiffer in the late 1950s, that seems to be effective without producing too many adverse effects. Dianol is a form of choline (2-di-methyl-aminoethanol) and appears to cross the blood-brain barrier quite easily.

Foods High in Choline

bean sprouts	liver (beef, pork)
beef	milk
egg yolk	peanuts
garbanzo beans	split peas
green beans	soybeans
lentils	

Foods High in VitamIn B$_5$ (Pantothenic Acid)

avocado	lobster
bean sprouts	mackerel
beef	mushrooms
chicken	peanuts
clams	pineapple
crab	salmon
egg	sardines
haddock	soybeans
lentils	watermelon
liver (beef, pork)	wheat germ

Foods High in Vitamin B$_1$ (Thiamine)

beef (heart, liver, kidney)	peas and other legumes
Brazil nuts	poultry
cereals	pumpkin
fish (mackerel, perch, red snapper)	soybeans
	sunflower seeds
lamb	wheat
liver (pork)	wheat germ
milk	yeast (brewer's)
oatmeal	

Learning and RNA

Ribonucleic acid (RNA), a basic structure of the blueprint for life, appears to be essential for learning processes. Several alleged memory enhancers, such as orotic acid, a substance found in milk, are in fact converted to RNA. Orotic acid combined with minerals such as magnesium, potassium, or calcium is available as a supplement in health food stores. High doses of RNA are needed to produce memory enhancement, and there is the added advantage that RNA helps cell protection against oxidizing agents, which cause cellular aging. Unfortunately, RNA does have some drawbacks:

1. Its acidity can cause stomach upsets.

2. RNA metabolism produces large amounts of uric acid, which can cause or aggravate gout and also precipitates into crystals that can deposit in the joints and kidneys.

Shopping for memory enhancers is like shopping for anything else: learn the facts or you will waste money. Some health food stores carry RNA, but unless a product contains more than 12 percent it is probably just yeast. Yeast contains about 6 percent RNA, but hardly any of it is available to the body because it is behind cell walls that our bodies cannot break down. The body, of course, makes RNA, and one way to stimulate RNA synthesis is to take vitamin B_{12}.

The Adrenaline Connection and Memory Enhancers

Norepinephrine, a chemical cousin of adrenaline (epinephrine), is another neurotransmitter that plays an important role in moods and behavior and may well be associated with memory. Its synthesis begins with the amino acid tyrosine, which is converted to dopamine. Excessive amounts of dopamine, a neurotransmitter in its own right, are associated with schizophrenia.

We know that amphetamines can cause psychosis, and we also know that amphetamines are triggers for the release of brain dopamine. In fact, some of the most successful antipsychotic drugs work by binding the dopamine receptors in the brain and therefore preventing their

Why Coffee Is a Stimulant

Most people know that caffeine and theophylline (active ingredients of coffee and tea) can help you to "wake up." Coffee is a "natural" substance belonging to a chemical group known as *methylxanthines*.

Methylxanthines inhibit the phosphodiesterase, the enzyme that destroys cyclic adenosine monophosphate (cAMP), which is the principal activator of most, if not all, neurotransmitters in the brain. So, anything that tends to lower phosphodiesterase levels will enhance neurotransmitter activities, and that is exactly what caffeine does.

Vitamin C (ascorbic acid) acts in the same way: it inhibits phosphodiesterase and increases cAMP levels in the brain. If not for the fact that taking a cup of vitamin C can cause diarrhea, we could easily substitute it for our morning coffee.

In spite of this, most orthodox psychiatrists continue to say that caffeine stimulates the brain but deny that vitamin C has any effect whatsoever, apart from preventing scurvy. So, whether you fancy coffee or a cup of vitamin C, you can rest assured that it will help your brain to function a little better, for a while at least.

---

activation by the transmitter. Vitamin C (ascorbic acid) and vitamin B_3 (niacinamide) are also said to have the same effect.

The principal dopamine enzyme, dopamine beta hydroxylase, depends on both calcium and vitamin C, which probably accounts for the observed calming effects of these nutrients. Dopamine is eventually converted to norepinephrine, which also plays a very important role in the control of human behavior and moods. Low levels of norepinephrine are closely associated with depression and an inability to think clearly.

ADRENALINE

Adrenaline (epinephrine) is the adrenal counterpart of the brain's own norepinephrine and is one of the most significant memory enhancers our body makes.

People learn best when they are motivated, alert, and stimulated. During the Second World War, German pilots were able to fly non-stop at night from Germany to England. This was no mean feat in those days, and it demanded superhuman powers of concentration. A captured Luftwaffe pilot was found to have been injected with an extract of a brain chemical known to stimulate the adrenal glands, which largely control how alert we are.

Research centers in the United States worked to reproduce this substance, adrenocortical stimulating hormone (ACTH), which stimulates the production and release of natural steroids. It also became clear that when the adrenal glands produced epinephrine (adrenaline), mnemonic abilities were enhanced significantly.

In the late 1970s, a brilliant series of experiments by James McGaugh, professor of psychobiology at the University of California, clearly showed that the brain's ability to memorize can be influenced by drugs that affect the levels of both epinephrine (adrenaline) and norepinephrine (noradrenaline).

Although only small amounts of these chemicals are found in the brain, the large amounts secreted by the adrenals during a state of excitement appear to be the primary factor in memory. Because adrenal secretions are the primary responses of the body to stress stimuli, it would seem that strong emotions act as an embalming fluid for memories. It is almost as if an event will not become part of our conscious experience unless adrenal hormones cry out "print it!" If emotions and chemicals are the "ink" of memory, then the complex circuitry of nerve cells and their myriad connections are the "paper" on which events are recorded.

Phenylalanine is a precursor, or source, of norepinephrine. This amino acid can be found in meat, cheese, or chocolate and is also available as an amino acid supplement. It is an excellent natural painkiller, antidepressant, and memory enhancer. Its only drawbacks are that it is very expensive and may elevate blood pressure in sensitive people. When used properly, it is probably the best natural antidepressant available today.

Tyrosine is another amino acid that produces norepinephrine. Levels of tyrosine in the brain are reliant on dietary levels of tyrosine, vitamin B_{12}, and magnesium.

Foods Containing Phenylalanine

almonds	egg
apple	herring
avocado	milk
baked beans	parsley
banana	peanuts
beef	pineapple
beet	soybeans
carrot	soy proteins
chicken	spinach
chocolate	tomato
cottage cheese	

Foods Containing Tyrosine

alfalfa	egg
almonds	fig
apple	herring
apricot	leek
asparagus	lettuce
avocado	milk
baked beans	parsley
banana	peanuts
beef	peppers (red, green)
beet	poultry
carrot	soybeans
cheese	spinach
cherries	strawberries
chicken	watercress
chocolate	watermelon
cottage cheese	yogurt
cucumber	

The Neuropeptides

The discovery of neuropeptides, small protein fragments that act as chemical signal modulators, has caused a flurry of activity among neurobiologists as they try to clarify the role of these chemicals in brain functions. Neuropeptides seem, at this stage, to have a dual role. They are capable of triggering complex behavioral responses when applied to the brain, and in most other parts of the body they act as local hormones, or regulators.

Vasopressin, a neuropeptide and an antidiuretic hormone produced by the pituitary gland, can increase memory when applied to the brain. A synthetic form of vasopressin found in nasal sprays has been

Foods to Think By

Foods, drugs, and several beverages have always been associated with creativity in one way or another.

Alcohol and fermented beverages have played a prominent role in the creative process for writers, notably Hemingway, Faulkner, and Fitzgerald, who all used alcohol extensively to enhance their creative moods.

Faulkner once said he could not even begin to write without a bottle of Scotch nearby, while the mathematician Poincaré found coffee essential to his work, and the English poet Housman found beer and tea to be necessary.

Chocolate can also be a powerful stimulant, probably because the brain uses one of its chemicals, phenylethylalanine, to manufacture norepinephrine.

An unusual chemical called *thujione*, a relative of nutmeg, is said to exert a powerful stimulating effect on the brain. A constituent of absinthe, this chemical is added in small quantities to vermouth and is a major component of cedar leaf oil.

Regardless of what you may need to think better, one thing seems clear: large meals make thinking more difficult, while fasting enhances the creative processes.

reported to restore memory to amnesia patients and to improve concentration ("Mind Foods," *Omni*, Jan. 1983, p. 40).

At this time, the biological significance of using the same chemical for apparently quite different purposes is not clear, but the field is one that promises many surprises.

Increasing Your Brain Power

Many nutritional scientists have found that certain vitamins enhance brain function. I have often seen an improvement in mental ability as a result of treatment that involved the use of vitamins for other problems.

In order to function properly, brain cells, like all body cells, need to be constantly supplied with molecules derived from the nutrients in the food you eat. Because the brain cells' functions involve thinking, anything that results in less than optimal nutrition for the brain cells will result in less than optimal thinking by the brain.

- It has been discovered that **vitamin C** interacts with an enzyme called *phosphodiesterase*, which reduces the brain levels of cyclic AMP and therefore raises all brain cell responses to normal. Vitamin C is abundant in peppers, tomatoes, and citrus fruits.

- It has also been found that **choline**, or **lecithin**, is essential for proper brain cell communication, attention span, and motor coordination. This substance has also been associated with improved mental ability. Choline is found in whole grains; beans (particularly soybeans); cold-pressed oils such as sunflower, safflower, and sesame; and lecithin granules and capsules.

- **Vitamin B$_5$** (pantothenic acid) has been found to help children with learning difficulties.

- **Vitamin B$_6$** (pyridoxine) is essentially linked with the formation of several important brain chemicals and the integrity of the nervous system. This vitamin has been reported to produce mental improvement in children suffering from a variety of problems ranging from autism to hyperactivity.

- **Copper** tends to overexcite brain cells. **Zinc** is capable of counteracting the action of copper in the body and therefore minimizes copper's negative effects on the brain.

- **Zinc** deficiencies have been linked with autism.

- Low levels of vitamins have been linked, in general, with excess activity of the nervous system and an inability to concentrate.

- **Gamma-aminobutyric acid** (GABA) helps cells in different parts of the brain to communicate with each other. It is made in the brain from glutamic acid, an ordinary amino acid present in food. This conversion, however, is only possible with the help of vitamin B_6.

- **Glutamic acid** also picks up excessive ammonia from the brain cells. A form of glutamic acid called L-glutamine is particularly effective in this function. It has been shown to improve thinking, clear the brains of alcoholics, reduce foggy minds during hangovers, and improve early morning alertness.

- Norepinephrine, another brain neurotransmitter associated with brain alertness, is derived from the amino acids **tyrosine** and **phenylalanine**. Brain levels of norepinephrine are related to the dietary levels of tyrosine, vitamin B_{12}, and magnesium.

- **Ribonucleic acid** (RNA) is now believed to be the stuff of which memory is made. RNA is plentiful in eggs, fish, and other high-protein foods. However, the body needs vitamin B_6 to break down the proteins into amino acids, and vitamin B_{12} and inositol to make RNA.

- Reduced thinking ability can be the effect of peroxidation and free radicals. **Vitamin E, vitamin A, carotene,** and **vitamin C** help to protect brain cells against this.

- Antioxidants also help against free radicals. There are several amino acids and nutrients that are important: para-aminobenzoic acid (PABA), L-cysteine, taurine, ginkgo, magnesium, zinc, ginseng, garlic, methionine, and selenium.

- The metabolic rate of the whole body is regulated by a gland called the *thyroid*. The functions of this gland are enhanced by kelp and iodine.

MOOD SWINGS: HOW TO CONTROL THEM

CHAPTER 2

Moods are very subjective. What may be considered a neurotic outburst by one person may be a show of normal temperament by another. However, an inability to keep an emotional even keel in the face of life's daily waves, a constant switch between anger and love, hyperactivity, and depression can reach dramatic proportions in some individuals.

There are many reasons for having uncontrollable mood swings. Some reasons are simple and obvious, and others are obscure and very, very complex. So let us look at some of the possible causes for up-and-down moods and then look at some of the ways to control them without the use of drugs. The diagnostic and treatment methods outlined are used at the Complementary and Environmental Medicine Center in Sydney.

How Histamine Affects Your Moods

Histapenia and *histadelia* refer to a condition in which there is either too much or too little histamine in the brain. Both conditions can alter the way we behave. The body has two separate receptors for histamine: H_1, which is involved in the classic histamine allergic reactions, such as headaches; and H_2, which is a brain receptor.

EXCESSIVE HISTAMINE LEVELS

Histadelics are people with excessive histamine levels who often have a large capacity for alcohol and other drugs. *Histadelics* tend to have a high libido and are subject to periodic and deep bouts of depression. Although their bouts of depression may be short and relatively infrequent, when they do occur histadelics may entertain suicidal thoughts. They seem to need less sleep than most people, tend to be somewhat obsessive, and are strangely sensitive to physical pain. They often suffer low or fluctuating blood-sugar levels (hypoglycemia) and adrenal exhaustion (hypoadrenocorticism) because they tend to be fast metabolizers. These conditions appear to fluctuate widely, from week to week, and even from day to day. They tend to have some allergies or intolerances that are often well masked, and they are prone to headaches or migraines. Histadelics tend to have good teeth because they salivate a lot and tend to have bad stomachs because they are tense.

Blood tests can be used to determine histamine levels. A differential white cell count will indicate a basophil count. Normal range for basophils is somewhere between 10 and 140. A high figure indicates high histamine levels.

Other common tests used to indicate histamine levels are the mean corpuscular volume (MCV) and the mean corpuscular hemoglobin content (MCHC). The MCV measures how large red blood cells are, and the MCHC measures how much hemoglobin the red blood cells contain. A low MCV with a high MCHC points to the possibility of high histamine levels.

TREATMENT

The main thrust of orthomolecular treatment is aimed at reducing histamine levels. Methionine, an essential amino acid, tends to methylate histamine and deactivate it. Pangamic acid, also known as calcium pangamate or vitamin B_{15}, is also useful in reducing histamine levels, as is a diet high in cabbages, especially the Chinese red variety.

Vitamin C has a natural antihistamine effect, while calcium tends to help the release of histamine.

Pharmaceutical drugs such as Dilantin (only available by prescription) can be used, because they interfere with vitamin B_{12} and folic acid metabolism. Vitamin B_{12} enhances the production of histamine. However, natural therapists prefer not to use drugs, although it is sometimes necessary to do so to bring about fast results. In this case, the drug should be used for only a couple of weeks, gradually reduced, and then eventually withdrawn after a month or so.

Taking large amounts of supplements, such as tyrosine, phenylalanine, or pantothenic acid, may, however, be counterproductive because they tend to stimulate the nervous system, which is already overstimulated by the excessive histamine.

A thorough check for food intolerances or allergies is mandatory, and fasting will generally help, since histamine synthesis is slowed down by a lack of proteins.

LOW HISTAMINE LEVELS

Histapenics are people who suffer from a deficiency of the neurotransmitter histamine and have fluctuating moods as a result. Their mean corpuscular volume tends to be high, pointing to a deficiency of

Foods Containing Methionine

apple	garlic
beef	ham
Brazil nuts	liver
Brussels sprouts	milk
cabbage	pineapple
cauliflower	pork
chicken	sardines
chives	soy
cottage cheese	soybeans
egg	watercress
fish	yogurt

Foods High in Vitamin B$_{15}$ (Pangamic Acid)

almonds	rice bran
apricot kernels	rice shoots
liver	yeast (brewer's)

dietary or absorbed vitamin B_{12} and folic acid. A routine blood test will often also show a low basophil count (usually well below 10).

Although histapenics appear to have rapid mood swings, the tendency is usually on the down side. They are likely to be daydreamers, often out of touch with reality and generally are low achievers who show little productivity in their work or chosen career. They are easily frustrated and become quite irritable, and as soon as they are under stress, they become physically tired and easily depressed. They get drunk on very small amounts of alcohol and are easily affected by most drugs. They generally seem to need a lot of sleep. They have a lowish sex drive, have a slow metabolism, and can generally tolerate pain quite easily. They tend to be somewhat paranoid and often think the world is against them.

TREATMENT

Treatment for histapenics involves large doses of vitamin B_{12} to increase histamine levels. Large doses can be given by injections or taken orally. Injections of vitamin B_{12} can cause problems with people who are allergic or hypersensitive to yeast, and so care should be taken with this treatment. Vitamin B_{12} taken orally seldom produces any problems. The B_{12} Plus tablets have been found to be very effective.

Folic acid seems to increase the effects of estrogen and may be contra-indicated in some patients with the following history: mammary tumors; hyperestrogenism; and a type of premenstrual syndrome characterized by often clotty and excessive menstrual blood (menor-rhagia), breast swelling and tenderness, lethargy rather than irritability during the premenstrual phase, and a tendency to retain a great deal of fluid (see Chapter 7 on premenstrual syndrome).

More recent research also indicates that people with the above history should not take yeast supplements, as they may be allergic to yeast or have a yeast infection. For persons not intolerant of or allergic to buckwheat, yeast is a valuable source of rutin, which prevents the breakdown of histidine. (Rutin, mixed with other vitamins, can also be taken in tablet form—check with your local health food store.)

Niacin, not niacinamide, should be given to help convert histidine to histamine, and a thorough check for wheat, gluten, and grain sensitivity should be made by a food provocation test. Other tests for detecting food sensitivities are not as reliable as the food provocation test. RAST tests measure only immunoglobin E reactions, and most food allergies are mediated by other immunoglobins. The cytotoxic test is very old and has proven to be unreliable and not reproducible. More up-to-date tests, such as the ALCAT test, are now available. However, such tests can be very costly and are inferior to the food provocation test.

Foods High in Vitamin B$_{12}$ (Cyanocobalamine)

beef (kidney, liver)	pork (hearts, liver)
cheese (cheddar, cream)	prunes
chicken	salmon
egg yolk	sardines
herring	shellfish
mackerel	tuna
milk	yogurt

Foods High in Folic Acid

almonds	orange
asparagus	peanuts
avocado	pecans
barley	plums
beef (heart, liver)	raisins
blackberries	rice
cottage cheese	spinach
dates	tuna
legumes	turkey
lettuce	walnuts
lima beans	wheat germ
mackerel	

Phenylalanine, tryptophan, and tyrosine may be helpful as depression is often connected with a deficiency of these neurotransmitters. My clinical experience has shown that tryptophan can worsen the symptoms of some psychiatric patients. If the underlying problem is a lack of norepinephrine, increasing serotonin (the product of tryptophan) will cause further imbalances of the ratio between the two neurotransmitters (serotonin from tryptophan and norepinephrine from tyrosine). If, however, the underlying problem is a deficiency of serotonin, tryptophan may be used successfully.

Vitamin B_5, or pantothenic acid, can also be a useful supplement because of its role in the transmission of nerve impulses in the brain and in helping the adrenal glands respond to stress.

In all cases, whether high or low histamine levels are suspected, a tissue saturation test for vitamin C should be performed in addition to the routine urine analysis carried out during the food allergy test.

Foods High in Niacin

avocado	potato
baked beans	raspberries
barley	rice
beef	salmon
broccoli	soy proteins
chicken	squash
clams	strawberries
fish (haddock, halibut)	tomato
liver	tuna
mushrooms	turkey
organ meats (liver, kidney)	watermelon
oysters	wheat
pork	yeast (brewer's)
peanuts	

Anxiety (LIAS) and Agoraphobia

THE CASE OF JOANNA X

Joanna, a 30-year-old business executive who travels all over the world as part of her job, came to see me some time ago.

"To put it quite bluntly, Dr. Vayda," she said, "I think I am about to get the sack. I am very good at my job and was promoted relatively early to a top buyer position about a year ago. After a few months of traveling, I began to experience episodes of what I call a foggy brain and anxiety. All of a sudden, and for no apparent reason, I would just be unable to think. Things that I would normally do almost without even thinking would be totally forgotten, or, quite abruptly, I would find myself almost incapable of carrying out the simplest task. I could not add up or make a decision about a particular line or even think coherently about what I was supposed to do. After a few such episodes, I began to feel fearful and often panicky—for no apparent reason.

"I would spend hours on end shaking and feeling something terrible was going to happen to me. I began to be afraid of leaving the hotel room—the only place, I may add, where I felt safe. I knew the feeling was somewhat similar to what I heard described as agoraphobia.

"I was not sick, yet I felt unwell. I didn't have a cold, a fever, or the flu, yet parts of my body began to ache in a subtle but disconcerting way. A number of doctors put me through every imaginable test but could only tell me I was perfectly healthy. I was told over and over again that it was all in my mind or from the stress of my job. Jet lag and premenstrual syndrome were blamed, as was the fact that I was unmarried, worked too hard, or did not have any children. It really boiled down to the particular personal beliefs of the attending physician. Yet in my own heart I knew something else was wrong. Although it clearly affected my brain, I also knew I was not mad or neurotic.

"I took a week off in Honolulu, sat on the beach, swam, sunbathed, and generally rested. I did not improve much, although I felt less anxious. So much for the suggestion that I just needed a holiday. And anyway, I had been working for only a couple of months since my last break—hardly the stuff to put a healthy 30-year-old out of action. By the end of the week I convinced myself there was nothing I could do about it and went back to work. I am now back in Australia, and I am afraid that, unless I can find a way to calm down, I will have to take tranquilizers or risk getting the sack."

I asked Joanna if she participated in any sport. She told me that she usually played some tennis, but since being unwell she found she lacked the energy. "Anyway," she added, almost as an after-thought, "whenever I exert myself physically I feel the symptoms either begin or, if already present, get worse, particularly the anxiety." For me, this last statement clinched the diagnosis.

A short series of questions established that Joanna drank alcohol moderately, yet daily, and that she drank about four or five cups of coffee and perhaps two cups of tea each day. Her diet includ-ed a fair amount of sweets, and she often resorted to fast-food snacks, which consisted primarily of refined carbohydrates. Her medical history revealed the fact that she had suffered a bout of hepatitis a few years ago.

I reassured Joanna that she was not likely to be allergic to any-thing and that allergies had nothing to do with her condition. Joanna was not mentally ill, although she did exhibit and experi-ence the symptoms of anxiety neurosis, but she did not need to take a single tranquilizer. However, within a few months she was back to her normal self.

You see, Joanna was suffering from lactate-induced anxiety syn-drome (LIAS), a condition that may be responsible for between 20 and 50 percent of all anxiety cases. Joanna's impaired liver was not able to perform some of the key steps in the biochemical chain that breaks down carbohydrates into glucose. Instead, she pro-duced abnormal amounts of a form of lactic acid called *lactate*. This natural chemical is a known panicogenic, which means it is capable of causing anxiety, or panic, in susceptible individuals.

Anxiety has different meanings for many people: irritable, nervous, fearful, panicky, touchy, excitable, moody, terrified, apprehensive.

These are all words commonly used to describe a state of mind that makes some people afraid to confront or cope with everyday tasks. Some people begin to sweat profusely at the thought of going to a job interview or meeting a new person, while others cannot even bear to get on a bus or go down to the corner shop. (In extreme cases, this condition is known as agoraphobia).

One symptom that is common in almost all cases of anxiety is a constant, or cyclic, lack of energy. Other signs include a rapid heartbeat; palpitations; a feeling of inner shakiness often accompanied by actual physical and visible shaking of the hands, limbs, or even the whole body; a feeling of tightness in the throat; muscular cramps; and moist palms.

Many sufferers experience mental confusion, unsteadiness, even dizziness, plus intermittent feelings of extreme fear and hopelessness, accompanied by a sense of impending doom. It is very common for such people to be labeled "neurotic" by friends, relatives, and sometimes even their own doctor.

On physical examination, someone suffering from anxiety will have elevated diastolic blood pressure. However, in cases where tiredness is a major symptom, blood pressure may be quite low. There is a ten-

Foods High in Vitamin B$_5$ (Pantothenic Acid)

avocado	lobster
bean sprouts	mackerel
beef	mushrooms
chicken	peanuts
clams	pineapple
crab	salmon
egg	sardines
haddock	soybeans
lentils	watermelon
liver (beef, pork)	wheat germ

dency toward muscular cramps, and heart rates tend to be abnormally fast. Invariably, people suffering from anxiety find it difficult to sleep, and they tire easily.

While some people with anxiety may have a history of psychiatric illness, many more have been classified as neurotic. A fair proportion of sufferers have a history of alcohol abuse, liver disorders, malabsorption and recurrent thrush, low or fluctuating blood-sugar levels (hypoglycemia), and environmental and food hypersensitivities or allergies. Breathing disorders are also common. Some studies have shown that most, if not all, such patients derive up to 75 percent of their calories from refined carbohydrates and sugars.

In many cases patients report a worsening of symptoms immediately after strenuous physical effort. They describe themselves, and are often referred to, as people who are on edge. Paradoxically, this kind of individual often has an overwhelming need for solitude and a lack of sensory inputs.

While it is true that in some cases of anxiety neurosis or agoraphobia the patient has an underlying personality disorder or psychological problem, there are many instances where the syndrome is due to biochemical abnormalities that are related to nutritional imbalances or deficiencies.

One of the most common nutritional imbalances is an excess of lactate. Lactate is the ionic form of lactic acid—a normal by-product of metabolism—which increases during physical activity and muscular exertion. Lactate can trigger a panic or anxiety attack, and if too much lactate is always present in the blood, the patient may well be in a constant state of anxiety.

Experiments have shown that in more than 90 percent of anxious people and some 20 percent of "normal" individuals, an intravenous injection of lactate will cause an immediate anxiety attack. Normally some of the circulating lactate is broken down to carbon dioxide and water and expelled from the body. An individual's capacity to break down lactate varies, and there are many reasons for an excessive buildup of lactate in the blood stream.

Digested starches, sugars, refined carbohydrates, and honey sorbitol or fructose (fruit sugar) are converted to glucose (blood sugar) in several biochemical steps. In one of these steps pyruvate is formed, and too much of this may be converted to lactate when the liver is not functioning very well or when there is a deficiency in some of the B vitamins, notably vitamin B_1 (thiamine), vitamin B_3 (niacin), and vitamin B_6 (pyridoxine), and minerals such as magnesium or zinc.

Pyruvate is also associated with vitamin B_{12}: a deficiency of vitamin B_{12} can cause pyruvate levels to increase dramatically. Increased pyruvate levels can cause blood-sugar levels to plummet, and the resulting hypoglycemia causes its own set of secondary symptoms, such as lethargy and mental confusion.

An interesting property of lactate is that it forms a bond with circulating calcium. It is this property that has led to the use of calcium supplements in the treatment of anxiety. Calcium binds excess lactate in the bloodstream and therefore reduces the possibility of a lactate-induced anxiety attack. Calcium supplements are used not to cure anxiety neurosis or agoraphobia but to prevent or avoid anxiety attacks altogether.

Another approach to treating anxiety is aimed at increasing liver function with the correct diet (often moderately high in proteins and some-

Foods High in Calcium

almonds	molasses
Brazil nuts	oysters
broccoli	salmon
cheese (cottage)	sardines
clams	sesame seeds
crab	soybeans
egg yolk	turnip greens
legumes	vegetables (dark green
liver (beef, chicken)	leafy ones)
mackerel	yogurt
milk	

times high in fiber) and supplements. Vitamin C powder is used in the form of calcium ascorbate partly because ascorbic acid increases the synthesis of cyclic AMP, which stimulates the liver's uptake of lactate, and because the calcium will also tie up some of the excess lactate.

We never use bone meal because of possible heavy-metal toxicity, or calcium gluconate because it is poorly absorbed. Calcium lactate is not used because the calcium and lactate neutralize each other and there is insufficient free calcium to latch onto circulating lactate.

Calcium needs to be taken on an empty stomach at least two hours after a meal or one hour before. Tea, coffee, and other caffeine-containing preparations are not advised because they can increase the lactate-pyruvate ratio. Alcohol has a similar effect, and, in addition, it can jeopardize optimal liver functions. Drastic reduction in the consumption of fruit juices, honey, and other sources of fructose are recommended, as this sugar is quickly converted to lactate under anaerobic conditions.

A low-sugar, no-refined-carbohydrates diet, similar to the hypoglycemic regimen, is suggested for people suffering with LIAS. In addition, the patient is advised to sweat profusely (preferably in a sauna and not through exercise), because sweating is one way in which the body can rid itself of lactate.

After a trial period, the patient is reassessed for each specific symptom, and any symptom that persists is looked at again to determine if it has a different cause.

Hypoglycemia

Hypoglycemia is fluctuating blood sugar where the levels either drop to an abnormally low level or fluctuate widely or rapidly. Hypoglycemia is one of the most common causes of erratic behavior, especially if it causes unexplained fatigue, occasional dizziness, and a craving for sweets.

While hypoglycemia is no longer considered a disease, it is often associated with a junk-food diet that contains too many sugars. It can be triggered by white, brown, raw, or crystal sugar as quickly as it can be triggered by honey and molasses. In fact, refined carbohydrates, cakes, soft drinks, and even an excessive amount of dried fruit can cause the symptoms.

The underlying cause of this condition, which is really a symptom, is often an intolerance, hypersensitivity, or allergy to a common food, chemical, or environmental factor. In women, another very common cause can be candida infestation, often known as thrush or monilia.

We used to carry out a glucose tolerance test (GTT) over a period of several hours for diagnosis. The test is still performed today, but instead of sugar, different foods or chemicals are used to challenge the patient, while several different parameters are measured along with the fluctuations in blood-sugar levels.

Irrespective of the cause of hypoglycemia, we know that it can invariably be triggered by sugar. So the basis of the old hypoglycemic diet (no sugar, sweets, or refined carbohydrates plus small but frequent snacks) is still used. The actual foods in the diet, however, depend on the individual's susceptibility. Some people may be placed on a high-protein diet, while others may be on a high-fiber diet, and others still on special regimens that eliminate particular foods.

Vitamins and mineral supplements are always tailored to the individual. If the hypoglycemic is depressed most of the time, vitamin B_5 will help a lot. If there is a great deal of anxiety and irritability, vitamin B_5 may make things worse. Zinc, vitamin B, vitamin C (in this case not calcium ascorbate), and other supplements are also given.

Because the liver is intimately involved in the storing of blood sugar, it is essential that liver functions are maximized with an appropriate diet and supplements and that total abstinence from alcohol is maintained.

Medical drugs that affect the liver should be used only if absolutely necessary and with the utmost care. Because stress influences both our immune system and our sugar metabolism, relaxation, meditation, and the avoidance of stressful situations are recommended.

Allergies and Candida (Thrush)

Allergies and candida are intimately interwoven, and, apart from causing the hypoglycemic syndrome, they can also be responsible for unbelievable mood swings. I have seen and treated thousands of patients whose emotional life has been restored to reasonable levels simply by detecting and then treating their unsuspected intolerances, allergies, or hypersensitivities. With candida, the problem is far more complicated.

Candida infection is usually noticed only if and when it affects the vaginal, oral, or anal area. Vaginal candidiasis, to give it a medical

Foods High in Zinc

beef (liver)	milk
bran	mushrooms
Brazil nuts	oatmeal
brown rice	oysters
crab	pork
egg	pumpkin seeds
grains	sunflower seeds
herring	tuna
kidney	veal
lamb	yeast (brewer's)

Foods High in Vitamin C (Ascorbic Acid)

alfalfa	kidney
banana	liver (beef)
berries (blueberries, goose-	oysters
berries, raspberries,	peppers (green, red)
and strawberries)	potato
Brazil nuts	spinach
broccoli	sweet potato
Brussels sprouts	tomatoes
cabbage	vegetables (green
cauliflower	leafy ones)
citrus fruit (lemons,	watermelon
oranges)	
guava	

name, causes a strong itch, sometimes a smelly discharge, and uncomfortable sexual intercourse.

Candida, the yeast fungus responsible for candidiasis, inhabits the mouth, throat, intestine, and genitourinary tract of most humans. It normally causes no problem and is a "silent partner." When our natural resistance is compromised, candida begins to proliferate and take over. Any weakening of the immune system by stress, poor diet, sickness, including HIV/AIDS, or the use of certain drugs can cause a candida overgrowth.

Candidiasis cannot usually be diagnosed by orthodox methods, so a thorough medical and nutritional history is essential. Candida overgrowth invariably causes a sensitivity (intolerance or allergy, if you like) to yeast and other molds or fungi. One of the most common mistakes made by well-meaning practitioners is to treat the condition without diagnosing and correcting the multiple allergies that are invariably present.

Symptoms and signs include premenstrual syndrome; craving for sweets, bread, cakes, and fermented, smoked, or pickled foods; abdominal distension; colitis; constipation; diarrhea; flatulence; headaches; depression; irritability; anxiety; sinusitis; asthma; cystitis; fatigue; joint pains or stiffness; fluid retention; skin problems; and an inability to lose weight despite many strict diets.

As the organism continues to grow, it changes from its normal yeast-fungal form, in which it causes the hypersensitivity and allergy, to a mycelial-fungal form, which produces rhizoids. Rhizoids are long, root-like structures that are able to penetrate the gut wall and break down the normal barriers between the intestine and the blood.

Because of the breakdown in the barriers, many compounds enter the circulation and cause allergic reactions. If these compounds penetrate the blood-brain barrier, they can produce symptoms that can be very easily mistaken for mental illness. These incompletely digested proteins (polypeptides) have even been known to mimic real neurotransmitters and play havoc with our moods.

Candidiasis, and its far-ranging systemic effects, needs to be carefully treated by an experienced orthomolecular practitioner. First the candida organism must be destroyed. This is achieved only with an antifungal preparation, such as Mycostatin, which must be carefully administered. At the same time, the organism is literally starved with a diet that is yeast-free and has no refined carbohydrates and sugars. The immunological resistance of each patient must be restored with a combination of supplements and attention to environmental factors.

Even after immune system restoration has been achieved, and it can take anywhere from a few weeks to many months, the patient must be carefully monitored (via challenge tests) for any residual allergies. Then a variety of probiotics, such as *Lactobacillus acidophilus*, should be used to foster the growth of bacteria in the gut that normally keep the candida organisms at bay.

Even after successful elimination of excessive candida, the intestinal mucosa should be restored with a diet high in fiber, oleic acid, and biotin (a B vitamin available in egg yolk and liver). If this type of diet is not possible because of a grain allergy, glucomannan is used instead. After this phase, several specially formulated supplements are used to help restore the intestinal mucosa. Garlic is often used in conjunction with these measures.

Unfortunately, after treating many hundreds of patients with olive oil, biotin, and a high-fiber diet, I have found that it does not work

What Happens When You Develop an Allergy?

When you develop an allergy, your body develops antibodies against the offending food or substance, and forever after, when antibody and allergen meet, a small explosion occurs in your body, and various chemical substances (such as histamine) are released. Your body aims to fight what it sees as the enemy, but in the process body tissues can become irritated or injured.

If the affected tissues happen to be in the lining of your air passages, you sneeze, cough, or develop sinusitis; if they are in the intestinal passages, your digestion suffers; if brain cells are thus affected, you develop psychiatric symptoms. Allergies are very problematic because you never know what guise they will take or what part of the body will be the innocent bystander that gets knocked down in the scuffle between antigen and allergen.

very often. The man who first proposed this program, Dr. J. Bland, says, "Although not entirely successful, this program has been helpful . . . employed to alleviate symptoms of chronic conditions." It is effective in chronic states, but it seldom seems to cure the underlying condition. While the changes to mycelial candida are slowed down, the excessive growth of fungal candida sets up a powerful intolerance and saps the immunological competence of the host.

A CASE OF CANDIDA ALLERGY

Melissa was plagued by recurrent ear infections, skin rashes, and sinusitis. She was experiencing terrible mood swings and severe premenstrual syndrome symptoms, especially depression. She had also had thrush a few times in the past five years.

Her doctor, a general practitioner with an interest in nutrition and alternative medicine, had diagnosed candidiasis and prescribed antifungals as well as a yeast-free diet. Melissa felt quite terrible after taking the medicine, but her doctor explained to her that this was probably a "die-off" reaction, which would last only a few days while her body killed off the offending organisms. Unfortunately, the symptoms persisted, and she was forced to abandon the treatment.

I explained to Melissa that this was not at all uncommon, as many of these so-called die-off reactions are, in fact, an allergic reaction to candida. The clue was that the symptoms persisted after the four or five days during which a die-off is likely to occur. In fact, a die-off reaction is often diagnostic evidence of fungi and mold allergies. I also explained to Melissa that treatment for a candida infection is quite different from that for a candida allergy.

Candida infections usually require the concurrent treatment of one's sex partner and often of any other individuals, such as children, who come into close daily contact with the sufferer.

Candida can cause infections as well as allergies. Allergies are caused by altering the immune system, and infections are caused by the release of toxins. Candida can cause both in one individual.

Such a situation can result in a variety of symptoms involving organs and glands anywhere in the body—even those remote from the areas infected by the organism. Candidiasis can be associated with foods, chemicals, environmental allergies, intolerances, or sensitivities, as well as dysfunctions of many glands, and therefore hormone and enzyme systems.

The symptoms of an allergy to candida are similar to those of allergies or intolerances to molds and fungi, with one exception: the so-called die-off reaction can last a lot longer and be so severe that it impedes treatment if an infection is present at the same time. That means that when treatment with antifungal begins, dying candida organisms are reabsorbed, and, because they change and release toxins, the symptoms become worse. If the patient is allergic to molds, the reaction will be even more severe and last longer.

In addition, treatment to desensitize or neutralize any allergy to molds, fungi, or candida may actually cause a reaction instead of alleviating the symptoms. It is, therefore, important to know if someone is allergic. If so, we often choose to separate any desensitizing or neutralizing drops to keep the molds out of them. Then, after the antifungals have done their job, either the vaccine for molds is added to the existing one or a new one is made up and administered. Another way to avoid this problem is to use homeopathic preparations for the allergies and the candida.

Of course, the knowledge of an existing allergy or intolerance to candida and molds is also helpful in monitoring the usefulness of the treatment. Sometimes people are treated with just a diet and supplements. This may or may not be enough. If it is not, the patient will have a reaction when the mold-desensitizing procedure is started. This is a clear sign that the infection has not yet been successfully treated. Then we have the choice of persevering with the original treatment for a longer period; changing the remedy being used, often to a homeopathic one; or using an antifungal, such as nystatin.

Because an allergy to candida often spreads to include sensitivities to many environmental molds and fungi, I arranged to have several mold plates placed in Melissa's home and asked the mycologists to analyze them. The report told me her bedroom was full of cladosporium, aspergillus, and penicillium and had a light content of several other molds and fungi.

At this point, we started to check Melissa's allergies. An immunoglobin E blood test turned out to be normal, but a skin scratch test showed her to be very sensitive to several molds and fungi, especially TOE (trichophyton-mix, candida, pidermophytoninguinaie), aspergillus, penicillium, cladosporium, and *Candida albicans*.

I explained to Melissa that she would have to be desensitized and would need to be particularly careful of mold exposure in both her environment and her food. She followed my advice and within a few weeks was free of her symptoms.

Why Are Allergies More Prevalent Nowadays?

- More and more of us survive birth.

- More and more of us are not breast fed and therefore miss the colostrum that helps to build the immune system.

- More and more of us eat a diet that is up to 50 percent manufactured, processed, and synthesized and is from an increasingly narrow range of ingredients. Both these factors are prime ways to encourage allergies.

- More and more of our food contains substances that people cannot digest, such as wheat, sugar, and caffeine.

- More and more pollutants are appearing in everything from your favorite aftershave to the fertilizer used to grow your vegetables. City water may contain up to 200 chemicals!

- More and more materials we place next to our body or use in the house are by-products of petrochemical hydrocarbons, which are highly allergenic substances. So our homes, offices, cars, and shops contain more and more potential allergens.

To reduce your chances of becoming susceptible to many of these allergens, try to avoid synthetic materials, denatured and processed foods, and chemical contaminants and try to live the natural life as much as you can.

Obviously not everyone with mood swings, irritability, anxiety, fatigue, and skin and weight problems will have candida, hypoglycemia, excessive histamine, or a deficiency of ionized calcium. However, the prevalence of these conditions warrants a full analysis before toximolecular medicine is allowed to step in with powerful psychiatric drugs, addictive tranquilizers, and other toxic medications.

MOOD SWINGS, TRANQUILIZERS, AND NATURAL ALTERNATIVES

CHAPTER 3

I have been practicing nutritional medicine and psychiatry for almost a quarter of a century. During that time I have treated thousands of patients who have suffered from mental or emotional illnesses. Rarely if ever have I seen anyone who has been cured by taking tranquilizers.

I have, however, seen patient after patient whose life has been ruined by becoming addicted to these drugs. In addition, I know of hundreds of people who, once they decide to stop taking tranquilizers, suffer withdrawal symptoms more severe than those that caused them to seek help in the first place.

In my clinical practice I have successfully helped, advised, and even cured many people whose alleged mental problems were, in fact, rooted in biochemical imbalances, such as allergies or physical illness, that responded admirably to dietary anticandida regimens or precursor (amino acid) therapy.

What Are Tranquilizers? How Do They Work?

There are literally hundreds of pharmaceutical and natural tranquilizers taken by millions of people all over the world in an attempt to relieve what is generally known as nervous tension.

Tranquilizers are divided into two categories: minor and major tranquilizers. Minor tranquilizers are usually used for the relief of simple anxiety, muscle tension, and sleeplessness and sometimes to buffer the withdrawal from illicit drugs or alcohol. Major tranquilizers are reserved for people who, in the opinion of the prescriber, suffer from a psychiatric problem. Examples of the latter are schizophrenics, manic-depressive psychotics, and those with bipolar depression (also known as manic depression).

In addition, some of these drugs are short-acting, which means they produce an effect rather quickly but the effect is short-lived. In other words, you are unlikely to feel the effects of these medications one or two days after taking them. Some other tranquilizers are medium-acting or long-acting.

Millions of Americans, the majority of them women, take tranquilizers and other mood-altering drugs without quite knowing what they are or why they are taking them. Few people realize that in many if not all cases, tranquilizers are habit forming, cause side effects, and do not work at all after a few months. For all practical purposes, they are simply legal and socially acceptable drugs of addiction.

Anyone wishing to give up tranquilizers should be aware that some drugs in all of the above groups have a short life in the body, while others have a much longer life. Once again, this seemingly baffling differentiation has a simple meaning: in order to give up something, one must decide whether to cut down gradually or stop suddenly. Drugs that linger in the body for a long time need a very different timetable that those than are short-acting if one is to avoid, or at least minimize, the withdrawal effects.

There is a great deal of confusion as to what tranquilizers can and cannot be used for. Most people do not realize that some sleeping pills are, in fact, tranquilizers taken in large doses at bedtime.

Many people who take tranquilizers do not really understand what they are, what they can and cannot do, and what their long-term effects are. Even fewer people know how to give up tranquilizers once they have taken them and whether or not there are any natural, safe alternatives.

The effects of medications collectively banded under the umbrella term *tranquilizers* are not to create tranquillity by calming a troubled mind.

Tranquilizers tend to suppress the whole personality of the long-term user and, at best, act only as a filter through which daily events are perceived as less threatening. It is to be clearly understood that any event that is perceived as stressful, such as disappointments, arguments, or any kind of conflict, will undergo this "filtering" action irrespective of whether the individual would normally be able to cope with it.

In this way, the person taking the tranquilizers does not have the possibility of adjusting to the situation and is, therefore, denied any opportunity to learn to cope with what may well be a perfectly normal, everyday event.

Most people are prescribed tranquilizers because they have stresses in their lives with which they have difficulty coping. These stresses may be emotional, such as problems at home or work, problems with money, phobias and insecurities, or any number of factors that impact our lives. There are also physical, biochemical, and nutritional stresses, which include allergies, chemical sensitivities, severe premenstrual tension, candida infections, and postviral syndrome.

Because life is so stressful and people are often unwell without knowing exactly why, many tend to abuse tranquilizers to the point where they become addicted to them. In fact, the situation in America is so bad that we are regarded as a nation of pill poppers with serious drug problems.

Addiction Versus Withdrawal

Tranquilizers are supposed to calm you down; they are "anxiolytic," which is a medical term for antianxiety. Because some doctors still believe that most people suffering from depression are also anxious, they often prescribe tranquilizers. In fact, there is no evidence that tranquilizers are of any use against depression, and many depressed people who take tranquilizers end up committing suicide.

What symptoms are likely to prompt a doctor to prescribe tranquilizers? Here is a list of the most common ones: excessive sweating, panic attacks, palpitations, inability to sleep, shakiness, pins and needles, fearfulness, perceptual distortions, lack of concentration, lack of confidence, and phobias.

As I said earlier, and as all medical textbooks tell us, tranquilizers should be used for only a short time. However, often people take them for months, even years on end, and when they try to stop, they find they cannot because they suffer withdrawal symptoms. They have become addicted.

What are the withdrawal symptoms that keep people taking their tranquilizers? Here is a short list of withdrawal symptoms: excessive

Analgesic (Painkiller) Cough Suppressant

Name: Codeine

Short-term effects of an average dose: Masks pain by creating mental clouding, drowsiness, and, in some cases, mild to extreme euphoria

Narcotics

Names: Heroin, morphine, opium, methadone

Medical uses: Analgesics; methadone (used for heroin addiction)

Short-term effects of average dose: Masks pain by creating mental clouding, drowsiness, and mild to extreme euphoria. In contrast, some users experience nausea, vomiting, and an itching sensation. Methadone's effects last considerably longer (24 to 36 hours, compared with two to four hours.

Short-term effects of large dose: Same as average dose but of greater intensity; insensitivity to pain is enhanced; a dreaming state of relaxation but with total awareness is induced. In some cases there is a paradoxical effect of increased energy and mental clarity. Overdoses produce unconsciousness, slow and shallow breathing, cold and clammy skin, and a weak but fast pulse rate and may cause death. Also when mixed with other depressants, narcotics may cause death.

Long-term effects of chronic use or abuse: Physical addiction, lethargy, weight loss, difficulties with erection and ejaculation, and a loss of libido sweating, panic attacks, palpitations, inability to sleep, shakiness, pins and needles, fearfulness, perceptual distortions, lack of concentration, lack of confidence, nightmares, hallucinations, and convulsions.

No, this is not a misprint. The symptoms that cause someone to be prescribed tranquilizers are very similar to those that he or she will experience when trying to stop taking them!

Withdrawal symptoms: Restlessness, irritability, tremors, anorexia, panic, chills, sweating, cramps, watery eyes, runny nose, nausea, vomiting, and muscle spasms

Barbiturates

Common trade names: Amytal, Nembutal, Phenobarbital, Seconal

Medical uses: Sedation, relief from tension, anesthetic

Short-term effects of average dose: Used recreationally, these drugs are a little like alcohol but without the calories. They produce mild intoxication, loss of inhibition (users could become sexually aggressive), decreased alertness, decreased muscle coordination, relaxation, and sleep.

Short-term effects of large dose: All the effects of a lower dose will be accentuated with the addition of slurred speech, shallow and slow breathing, cold and clammy skin, weak and rapid heartbeat, and hangover feelings. Unconsciousness can move beyond sleep to coma and eventually death.

Long-term effects of chronic use or abuse: Sleepiness; confusion; irritability; severe withdrawal sickness with symptoms such as anxiety, insomnia, tremors, delirium, convulsions, and occasionally leading to death. Tolerance to sedatives increases, so one may need to take larger doses to obtain the same effect. Unfortunately, tolerance to a lethal dose does not increase, so that one may accidentally increase the dose to fatal levels.

Gluthetimide containing medications are similar to barbiturates, but because it is longer acting, the effects of an overdose are more difficult to reverse; they can be fatal.

People who have been taking tranquilizers for a while may decide to stop taking them. However, when they start to feel sick, to shake visibly, to experience anxiety attacks, or to become so fearful that they cannot leave home, they go back to their doctor and are often prescribed larger doses of the tranquilizers that are causing their withdrawal

Minor Tranquilizers

Long acting: Bromazepam, chlordiazepoxide, colbazam, chlorazepate dipotassium, diazepam, flunitrazepam, flurazepam, nitrazepam. Some common brand names are Librium, Tranxene, Valium. (These are the international names or the names for the actual active chemical ingredients, *not* brand names. The same chemical can have different brand names in different countries, and there can be several variants of the same chemicals. For example, Benzodiazepine is a general group of tranquilizers, of which diazepam is one. The common brand name for this is Valium.)

Medical uses: Relief from anxiety, muscular tension, and the symptoms of alcohol withdrawal

Short-term effects of average dose: Mild sedation, a sense of well-being, and an increased ability to cope. May cause headaches and in rare cases can have a paradoxical effect of increasing anxiety and hostile behavior.

Short-term effects of large dose: Drowsiness, blurred vision, slurred speech, and stupor. If mixed with alcohol, can cause suppression of breathing and even death.

Long-term effects of chronic use or abuse: Impairment of sexual functions, confusion, irritability, and severe withdrawal sickness, which can appear several days after intake has stopped. Tolerance to sedative effect increases, so one may need to take larger doses to obtain the same effect.

Withdrawal symptoms: Anxiety, insomnia, tremors, delirium, convulsions, and occasionally death

Medium acting: Aprazolam, Lorazepam, Oxazepam, Lormentazepam, Temazepam. They have the same advantages and disadvantages as the long-acting tranquilizers.

symptoms. The next inevitable step is that the patient becomes totally dependent on the drugs and remains on them full time.

Because the symptoms experienced by patients when they try to stop taking tranquilizers can be quite severe, many people give up and continue taking them. However, the incidence and severity of withdrawal symptoms can be greatly reduced by following a well-planned program that uses natural alternatives and other supportive therapy.

The Tranquilizer Cycle

If you are taking or are thinking about taking tranquilizers, you should be aware of a few facts:

- Doctors often prescribe drugs, such as Valium, Oxazepam, Diazepam, Nitrazepam, Temazepam, Flunitrazepam to people who are worried, sad, panicky, or unable to sleep.

- These states are often caused by things such as divorce, grief, domestic violence, a boring or overdemanding job, money problems, or any number of other physical stresses on your body.

- On some occasions, taking tranquilizers may help you to get through a crisis situation; however, taking them regularly will not resolve your marriage, pay your rent, or calm down an aggressive partner.

- Tranquilizers block out your feelings. Without feelings like anger, anxiety, or sadness, you are less likely to try to do something about resolving your problems and overcoming the crisis.

- Tranquilizers make your problems appear a little further away, but they can also make you feel listless, affect your coordination, and interfere with your ability to think clearly and therefore solve any problems!

- The longer you take tranquilizers, the less effect they have because your body builds up a tolerance to the drug. So the only way you are able to keep calm or sleep easily is by taking more.

- Eventually you find that you cannot function very well without tranquilizers and you are suffering from a dependency. In short, you have become an addict.

Natural Tranquilizers

As we have seen in the earlier part of this chapter, there are many reasons why tranquilizers are prescribed. Before any medication—natural or otherwise—is prescribed, it is essential to find out the cause of the problem and whether tranquilizers will benefit your condition.

There are a number of natural nutrients known as health supplements that can be taken instead of pharmaceutical tranquilizers. In many cases these natural alternatives are effective and have few, if any, side effects. Like all medications, they need to be prescribed by a competent therapist who is thoroughly familiar with any possible problems that may be encountered.

Nowadays, there is an amazing array of supplements, such as vitamins, minerals, and amino acids, available in health food shops. Each one has a different claim: to cure this or that, to make you slim forever, or to keep you free from heart disease.

It is no wonder that many people are confused and disillusioned about what to expect from some of these natural alternatives. There is an increasing number of people who take supplements hoping that they will provide a miracle cure for their ailments. Mental and physical health can at best be helped by supplements; it cannot be found in them!

Due to unsatisfactory results from these supplements, people often consult nutritional therapists to check that they are taking the right supplement and the right dose and that the primary cause of the problem has not been masked by their symptoms.

Following are some of the natural alternatives to tranquilizers. However, it must be stressed, once again, that any supplements for any type of mood disorder should be taken only under professional supervision.

PHENYLETHYLALANINE

One of the body's natural antidepressants is phenylethylalanine. This is a chemical substance derived from phenylalanine, a common amino acid found in many foods.

Phenylalanine is used by the brain to make norepinephrine (noradrenaline) and to slow the breakdown of the natural opiates (endorphins and enkephalines), which are responsible for, among other things, lowering the sensation of pain. Phenylalanine is sold as a supplement in the form of DL-phenylalanine (DLPA). DLPA may revolutionize the treatment of depression and intractable pain because it can be a very successful method for the nutritional control of chronic depression and some types of pain.

Health professionals, pain treatment clinics, and scientific research papers have reported dramatic results in patients with chronic depression; acute premenstrual syndrome; and severe, acute, and chronic pain conditions, including rheumatoid arthritis, back pain, migraines and headaches, postoperative pain, and neuralgia.

Phenylalanine is an essential amino acid that exists most commonly in high-protein foods, and in two forms called D and L. We can metabolize and utilize it and its by-products quite easily. It is nontoxic and has been found to be ten times less toxic than vitamin C.

DLPA analgesia requires anywhere from two to 14 or more days to develop, but its effects are long-lasting. After initial treatment, the patient may need to take DLPA only a few days (typically about seven) every month. It works in what is probably the ideal way, by intensifying and prolonging the body's natural painkillers, endorphins and enkephalines.

About ten years ago it was discovered that the human brain synthesizes a group of hormones with properties quite similar to those of morphine and opium. Appropriately, these were first called "the brain's own opiates" and were found to follow the activation of pain signals. These endorphin hormones are part of a natural built-in

"Regulations covering medications are much more lax than those covering pesticides. Valium, a common tranquilizer, is freely prescribed though it has a variety of side effects. These include drowsiness, fatigue, hypertension (high blood pressure), confusion, depression, constipation, headaches, hypoactivity (lassitude), hiccups, jaundice, nausea, skin rashes, slurred speech, tremors, blurred vision, anxiety, hallucinations and changes in salivation" (Dr. Allan Crawford, Director of Public Health, NSW *The Daily Mirror*, Sept. 14, 1982).

pain-relief system, which is activated in cases of extreme stress. It is the system responsible for the loss of pain sensation when people who have suffered traumatic injuries find that they remain unaware of the extent of their problems for several hours after the event.

One of the problems with painkilling hormones, and indeed with many natural chemicals, is that there is an array of enzymes in the body ready to destroy them. DL-phenylalanine inhibits several enzymes that destroy these natural painkilling hormones. The inhibition of these enzymes enables painkillers to affect their influence for a much longer period of time.

Another important consideration is that people suffering chronic pain and depression tend to have lowered levels of endorphins. DLPA is thought to restore endorphins to normal levels, thus allowing the normal painkilling effects of the brain chemicals to continue for longer periods.

One of the great advantages of using natural substances—rather than drugs—as painkillers is that the normal short-term signals of acute pain, such as the result of hitting your thumb with a hammer or touching boiling water, are not inhibited.

Foods Containing Phenylalanine

almonds	egg
apple	herring
avocado	milk
baked beans	parsley
banana	peanuts
beef	pineapple
beet	soybeans
carrot	soy proteins
chicken	spinach
chocolate	tomato
cottage cheese	

CONTRAINDICATIONS AND WARNINGS

While the use of a natural painkiller, such as phenylalanine, is still far safer than using pharmaceutical drugs, we must exercise extreme care when we start to tinker with the brain's chemistry.

At the Complementary and Environmental Medicine Center we have conducted a series of trials, and it appears that most of the claims for DLPA are indeed quite valid. We are, however, presently investigating its effects on behavior, and the preliminary conclusion is that it should be used with caution by people suffering from psychiatric disorders.

Dr. Richard Wurtman, a neuroendocrinologist at the Massachusetts Institute of Technology, suggests that a rise in phenylalanine may completely block the normal rise in brain serotonin levels that follows the ingestion of certain meals. Wurtman's study shows that when serotonin levels are prevented from rising, the brain is tricked into wanting more carbohydrates. One can only speculate at this point on the possible disruption in sleep patterns and mood changes that may occur because of this.

DLPA, and indeed *any* preparation containing phenylalanine, should not be taken by people suffering from phenylketonuria (PKU). It should not be taken during pregnancy, and people suffering from hypertension are advised to take it *after* instead of *before* meals (as it should normally be taken).

MAGNESIUM

Excessive nitrogen (fertilizers), phosphorus (soft drinks), copper (water pipes), and iron (through excessive consumption of red meat or unnecessary iron supplements or vitamin-mineral pills that contain iron) can cause an imbalance or deficiency of magnesium.

When magnesium levels are too low, the nervous system becomes easily irritated. At some stage, an individual will experience feelings of disorientation and may even have convulsions. Muscular twitching is a common symptom and can be reversed by the administration of magnesium.

Magnesium can be such a powerful peripheral nervous system depressant that excessive doses can cause flaccid muscles and even a degree of anesthesia. Patients with chronic insomnia, nervous tension, anxiety, and muscular tension have been repeatedly found to have low levels of magnesium in their blood.

The calming effects of magnesium have also been observed in animals, thus counteracting claims of placebo influence. Dr. Jerry Aikawa of the University of Colorado Medical Center treated 41 thoroughbred horses, two of which were known to be quite edgy. An analysis of the horses' blood showed that almost all the nervous ones had low blood magnesium levels. Once this mineral was added to their diet, the animals calmed down considerably, showing that magnesium can be an effective tranquilizer.

Foods High in Magnesium

almonds	lima beans
apricots, dried	molasses
avocado	oatmeal
baked beans	peaches
barley	peanuts
beef	peas
Brazil nuts	pecans
carrots (raw)	pork
cashews	potato
chicken	rice
citrus fruits	sesame
corn	soybeans
crab	tomato (raw)
dates	vegetables (dark green
fish (flounder,	leafy ones)
salmon, tuna)	wheat germ
lentils	

VITAMIN B$_1$ (Thiamine)

An article from the medical journal *Modern Medicine in Australia* described how a group of patients with symptoms such as sleeplessness, personality changes, aggressiveness, and irritability were found to be deficient in vitamin B$_1$. All the patients appeared to suffer from anxiety, and each of them responded to vitamin B$_1$ supplements with either a complete remission of symptoms or a marked improvement in their moods.

Vitamin B$_1$ acts as a coenzyme in the breakdown of carbohydrates by oxidizing pyruvic acid. If insufficient vitamin B$_1$ is available, pyruvic acid accumulates. This then becomes lactic acid, which is eventually turned into lactate.

The connection between lactate and anxiety is well documented. We know that high blood levels or an unusual sensitivity to this natural by-product of muscular exertion and sugars can cause anxiety attacks in susceptible people. A hereditary predisposition or early liver damage may cause some people to experience a continuous low-level background anxiety state.

This condition is known as lactate-induced anxiety syndrome (LIAS) (see page 29) and can often be treated successfully with large amounts

---

Foods High in Vitamin B$_1$ (Thiamine)

beef (heart, liver, kidney)	pork (liver)
Brazil nuts	poultry
cereals	pumpkin
fish (mackerel, perch,	soybeans
red snapper)	sunflower seeds
lamb	wheat
milk	wheat germ
oatmeal	yeast (brewer's)
peas and other legumes	

---

of supplementary calcium, vitamin B_1, and dietary manipulations to reduce pyruvic acid.

As well as being in excessive demand during periods of high carbohydrate consumption, vitamin B_1 is destroyed by food-processing methods such as heating and oxidation.

Alkalis also destroy vitamin B_1. People taking stomach alkalizers (antacids) often find that they become irritable and as a result experience an increase in stomach acidity, ulcer pains, and abdominal discomfort. To compensate, they need more antacids or alkalizers, and a vicious circle is thus established. The next step can be mental confusion and depression.

Studies have shown that vitamin B_1 deficiencies in children may result in lowered IQ levels (H. Guthrie, professor of nutrition, Pennsylvania State University, *Nutrition* C. V. Mosby, St. Louis, 1975, pp. 259–320).

VITAMIN B$_{12}$ (Cyanocobalamine)

A deficiency of vitamin B_{12} is known to cause pernicious anemia. What some people do not realize is that vitamin B_{12} deficiencies are also associated with depression, neurosis, some forms of schizophrenia, and psychosis.

Low vitamin B_{12} levels, or histapenia, also cause a rise in pyruvic acid, and as we have seen, this can lead to increased circulating lactate and a state of anxiety. The similarity with vitamin B_1, however, ends there.

Foods High in Vitamin B$_{12}$ (Cyanocobalamine)

beef (kidney, liver)	pork (hearts, liver)
cheese (cheddar, cream)	prunes
chicken	salmon
egg yolk	sardines
herring	shellfish
mackerel	tuna
milk	yogurt

Any of the following factors can contribute to a vitamin B_{12} deficiency: malabsorption, irritable bowel syndrome, low stomach acidity, excessive intake of antacids, prolonged strict vegetarian diet (vegan), and abuse of alcohol and/or several prescribed medications such as anticonvulsants.

People suffering from emotional disorders associated with vitamin B_{12} deficiency are known as histapenics because of the low levels of brain histamine (another neurotransmitter) this condition can cause. (For more information on histapenics, see page 25.)

VITAMIN B_6 (Pyridoxine)

Gamma-aminobutyric acid (GABA) is one of the neurotransmitters responsible for slowing down the chemical activity in the brain. Another neurotransmitter, glutamic acid, is responsible for exciting chemical activity.

Foods High in Vitamin B_6 (Pyridoxine)

avocado	milk
barley	molasses
beans	oranges
Brazil nuts	peanuts
carrot	peas
cheese	potato
cow's milk	prunes
crab	rice
egg	soybeans
fish (cod, halibut, herring,	spinach
mackerel, salmon,	sunflower seeds
sardines, tuna)	wheat bran
lentils	wheat germ
lima beans	whole-meal flour
liver (pork)	yeast (brewer's)
meat (beef, ham, pork)	

The manufacture of GABA is particularly reliant on ample supplies of vitamin B_6, and for this reason alone, vitamin B_6 is often useful as a tranquilizer.

However, another important factor also helps to explain the role of vitamin B_6 and its sedating effects. GABA (the inhibitory neurotransmitter) is made from glutamic acid (the excitatory neurotransmitter) in the presence of vitamin B_6. So if there is too little vitamin B_6, less GABA is made and the levels of glutamic acid rise, causing irritability of the central nervous system. However, if there is ample vitamin B_6, then a lot of GABA is made, which helps in sedating or calming down the brain.

At the same time, an excess of vitamin B_6 could deplete glutamic acid reserves to the point where proper excitation and hence perceptual functions of the nervous system may be impaired.

For more information on GABA, glutamic acid, and vitamin B_6, see page 10.

ZINC

Zinc has a calming effect on our nerves, and it also counteracts copper. Because of the widespread use of copper water pipes, many orthomolecular scientists feel that some individuals may suffer an overload of this mineral.

Foods High in Zinc

beef (liver)	milk
bran	mushrooms
Brazil nuts	oatmeal
brown rice	oysters
crab	pork
egg	pumpkin seeds
grains	sunflower seeds
herring	tuna
kidney	veal
lamb	yeast (brewer's)

Copper excites the nervous system, and this may be a reason why zinc is a very useful adjunct to the use of other natural tranquilizers.

Frozen vegetables are usually deficient in zinc. Some diets high in soya phytates may cause poor absorption of zinc. Alcohol abuse often creates a zinc deficiency, as does anything that tends to irritate the gut lining, including antibiotics, food allergies, and candida infestations.

VITAMIN C (Ascorbic Acid)

Most people associate vitamin C with the treatment or prevention of the common cold, influenza, and viral infections.

What is far less well known is the fact that although brain cells cannot make vitamin C, the concentration of this vitamin in the brain is higher than in any organ except the adrenal glands (the glands responsible for our responses to stress).

According to Dr. Abraham Hoffer, the pioneer of orthomolecular psychiatry, vitamin C is as active as some of the most powerful psychiatric medications in use today, simply because it acts as a dopamine receptor blocker.

Foods High in Vitamin C (Ascorbic Acid)

alfalfa	guava
banana	kidney
berries (blueberries,	liver (beef)
gooseberries, rasp-	oysters
berries, strawberries)	peppers (red, green)
Brazil nuts	potato
broccoli	spinach
Brussels sprouts	sweet potato
cantaloupe	tomatoes
cauliflower	vegetables (green
citrus fruit	leafy ones)
(lemons, oranges)	watermelon

Weight for weight, vitamin C does the job as effectively as Haldol, a dopamine antagonist widely used in the treatment of various forms of psychosis. High levels of dopamine in the brain are associated with aggressiveness, irritability, and a host of psychiatric conditions, such as schizophrenia.

In order for vitamin C to be effective in the brain, it has to be administered in huge doses so that at least a little will be forced to cross the blood-brain barrier.

VITAMIN B₃

There are two types of vitamin B_3, and each one has two names: niacin, also known as nicotinic acid, and niacinamide, also known as nicotinamide. In 1979, H. Mohler and his research group at Hoffman-La Roche (the Swiss pharmaceutical company responsible for Valium) discovered that nicotinamide is "a brain constituent with benzodiazepine-like activity . . . only nicotinamide showed the main neuropharmacological central effects characteristic of benzodiazepines although, because only 0.3 percent enters the brain, rather high doses are needed to elicit effects."

Benzodiazepine is the technical name for a group of chemicals that are used as minor tranquilizers, such as Valium. In order for vitamin B_3 to be effective in any central nervous system activity, it has to be administered in megadoses (hundreds of milligrams daily) so that at least a little will be forced, by mass action, to cross the blood-brain barrier.

Because nicotinamide has properties in common with Valium and barbiturates, it may be valuable as a general tranquilizer and as an anticonvulsant muscle relaxant, especially when administered together with magnesium.

These are some of the reasons why we sometimes prescribe megadoses of vitamin B_3. We know only too well that such high doses are needed to achieve any effect within the central nervous system.

Nicotinic acid (niacin) has quite different properties. It is very helpful as part of any treatment program for most schizophrenias, senility, and alcoholism but does not appear to have the same tranquilizing effects of niacinamide. This is probably because the naturally occurring form of vitamin B_3 in the human body is nicotinamide dinucleotide (NAD), which contains niacinamide, not niacin.

Foods High in Vitamin B$_3$ (Niacin)

anchovy	breakfast cereals
beef liver	mackerel
chicken	swordfish

DEPRESSION

Gloom and doom, sadness and madness, melancholy, the doldrums, languor, sorrow—depression has many names and is often described as the common cold of psychiatry. It is a very common problem, and, indeed, it is a rare individual who does not feel depressed at some time or another.

When psychiatrists speak of depression, however, they are talking about a clinical state of illness of which there are many types, and each kind of depression can have several symptoms.

The type of depression diagnosed will depend on the symptoms, an analysis of the patient's history, and perhaps some psychological or other tests. Then a suitable treatment is prescribed. Unfortunately, even though it sounds quite simple, it is not.

Depression can be unipolar (simple), the common garden-variety in which the sufferer is just—well, depressed, or bipolar. Bipolar depression is also known as manic depression, and a variation of it is called manic depressive psychosis (MDP). There is a variation of MDP known as seasonal affective disorder syndrome (SADS). There are also postpartum depression (PPD), endogenous depression ("from within" or "spontaneous"), and reactive depression.

Reactive depression means that when something unfavorable happens, you respond by being depressed. Although endless lists of such causes of reactive depression are regularly compiled by psychologists, the fact is that some things affect some people more than others; some people seem to shrug off adverse events, while others become depressed every time things do not run smoothly. Given the infinite variety of humans, this is entirely understandable. It is only when an individual fails to recover after the causative event has passed that such a permanently depressed state becomes a clinical illness.

Most of us find the many labels and terms used by psychologists and psychiatrists very confusing and not particularly helpful in finding the root of the depression.

Depression can be caused by almost anything: lowered immune responses; candida; alcohol abuse or overindulgence; vitamin B_{12} deficiency; an imbalance or deficiency of several minerals, nutrients, and amino acids; different kinds of anemia; malabsorption; hypoglycemia; or food allergies.

Depressed people can become obsessive or indolent, lackadaisical or compulsive, lazy or workaholics. In fact, the range of individual reactions to depression is almost as varied as human nature. The only thing they all have in common is the depression. There are, of course, some well-known causes for depression.

It is often the case that many people who suffer from depression are also overweight. The therapist must always try to assess if any particular individual is depressed because he or she is overweight or overweight because he or she is depressed. The fact is that the two seem to go hand in hand.

Special assessment tests, such as the Hoffer and Osmond diagnostic test, are very effective in detecting true clinical depression. Following are some of the reasons why depression can lead to weight gain and a discussion about some of the common causes of depression.

Touching, Tyrosine, Depression, and Weight Gain

Today we know that stress in general can cause the body's levels of noradrenaline (also called norepinephrine) to become exhausted. Low levels of noradrenaline are associated with depression. Using drugs that do not elevate noradrenaline levels will not alleviate this type of depression.

Therapists familiar with nutritional (orthomolecular) psychiatry also know that otherwise useful nutrients, such as vitamin B_6, tryptophan, and zinc, and high complex carbohydrate diets, such as vegetarianism and Pritikin, will not usually resolve this type of depression and may make it worse. Conversely, we know that whenever stress is a strong contributing factor in clinical depression, tyrosine is probably the treatment of choice.

Foods Containing Tyrosine

alfalfa	egg
almonds	fig
apple	herring
apricot	leek
asparagus	lettuce
avocado	parsley
baked beans	peanuts
banana	peppers (red, green)
beef	poultry
beet	soybeans
carrot	soy proteins
cheese	spinach
cherries	strawberries
chicken	watercress
chocolate	watermelon
cottage cheese	yogurt
cucumber	

Depression often, but not always, goes hand in hand with low blood pressure, low blood sugar, low thyroid functions (all of which tend to contribute to weight gain), and low adrenal gland functions.

Tyrosine can normalize blood pressure, stimulate the thyroid, and contribute to blood-sugar stabilization via adrenal support. Patients suffering with this kind of depression often crave many different types of foods, and while these may include sweets, there can also be a strong desire for cheese, chocolate and other tyrosine-containing foods.

If digestion is impaired, by low hydrochloric acid states or intestinal candidiasis, for example, dietary tyrosine is converted to tyramine. Tyramine stimulates the adrenal glands and causes further depletion of noradrenaline stores while at the same time depriving glands like the thyroid of needed tyrosine. The following diagram shows us this relationship.

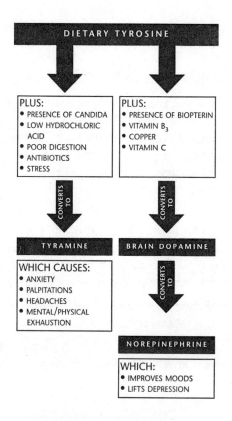

Tyrosine is one of the three aromatic amino acids, the other two being phenylalanine and tryptophan, that cross the blood-brain barrier. Levels of tyrosine in the brain depend somewhat on dietary intake. However, just taking tyrosine supplements is not enough to increase levels.

Tyrosine competes with other amino acids, especially the branched amino acids (leucine, isoleucine, and valine), to be transported from the blood to the brain. Along with tryptophan, the branched amino acids inhibit the brain's uptake of tyrosine. So tyrosine is more likely to be beneficial if taken on an empty stomach.

The metabolism of tyrosine depends on a form of folic acid (biopterin) and a type of vitamin B_3 (NADH) as well as copper and vitamin C. Once tyrosine reaches the neurons, it is converted to dopamine and then norepinephrine, which helps lift depression.

This last but crucial step, however, depends on the presence of an enzyme (tyrosine hydroxylase) at the presynaptic nerve ending. The availability of the enzyme, and therefore the output of useful norepinephrine, depends on the amount of electrical activity along the nerve.

When *anything* touches you, nerve impulses are transmitted from the point of impact to the brain. Therefore, chiropractic, osteopathy, massage, acupuncture, caressing, touching, or any physical contact will cause an increase of electrical nerve impulses. This will increase the amount of the enzyme tyrosine hydroxylase, which is necessary to produce the antidepressant neurotransmitter chemical norepinephrine.

In addition, tyrosine is the precursor of the thyroid hormone. Low thyroid function tends to go hand in hand with high estrogen and a lack of vitamin E. This combination makes for poor circulation, weight gain, a slow metabolism, and lack of libido.

There is very little tyrosine in cereals, grains, fruit, vegetables, or oils. The highest concentrations are to be found in wild game and yogurt.

Tyrosine tends to elevate blood pressure in people suffering with low blood pressure and lower it in those suffering with high blood pressure: it exerts an adaptogenic and normalizing effect.

THE CASE OF MARY X

Mary X was referred to me because she was suffering with depression, digestive disturbances, such as bloating and intestinal gas, as well as diarrhea and constipation. She was grossly overweight but denied overeating and was not particularly fond of sweets. She tended to be anxious, fearful, and somewhat shaky. Her mental state was one of confusion, and she described herself as "unable to cope." Her skin tended to be dry, her menstrual blood was often clotty, she suffered with recurrent skin rashes, her breasts became sensitive before her period, and she felt cold easily, always complaining of icy hands and feet.

Mary displayed many of the symptoms of hypothyroidism (low thyroid function). A basal temperature test confirmed this fact. The original diagnosis, made by the referring practitioner, had been of candida, and indeed, a yeast-free diet coupled with antifungal medications improved her skin and most of her digestive symptoms. However, she still had difficulties losing weight and was very depressed and somewhat anxious.

Mary was under a great deal of personal stress in her relationship, and her mother had recently passed away. A blood test confirmed that Mary had a mild yeast infection, but when I analyzed the results I discovered her immune system was working reasonably well and taking care of that situation.

I asked Mary to attend a competent masseur and suggested that she have a massage every day. I also told her to ask her partner to give her plenty of cuddles. Keeping the whole thing in a somewhat light vein, I discussed the matter with her partner and explained that Mary was not neurotic or in any way mentally ill but that she suffered from a number of biochemical and nutritional problems that could easily be overcome. I assured him she would soon be well and explained that his cooperation would make this happen much faster.

In addition to extra hugging and touching, Mary was prescribed supplements of tyrosine to be taken in the morning and again midmorning, always on an empty stomach. Within four weeks Mary had lost eight pounds, she was no longer depressed, and most of her anxiety was a thing of the past.

Tyrosine and Cancer

The idea that certain types of cancer need specific amino acids to thrive is not a new one. As far back as the 1960s, trials were carried out with low-phenylalanine diets in an attempt to "starve" cancer cells. Success with this treatment was less than hoped for.

There are certain forms of cancer, such as malignant melanomas and glioblastoma multiforma, in which the cancer cells are known to soak up tyrosine at a great rate. It would be prudent, therefore, not to use this amino acid under those circumstances unless the possible advantages clearly outweigh the potential risk.

CONTRAINDICATIONS AND WARNINGS

Tyrosine, like most aromatic amino acids, may be contraindicated in some types of schizophrenia. Orthomolecular practitioners are well aware of the contraindications of amino acid supplementation in psychosis and assess each patient carefully before administering megadoses.

Psychiatric assessment tests, such as the Hoffer and Osmond diagnostic test, coupled with a thorough medical history and details about the effects of previous medications are all carefully considered. In some cases, of course, it is quite reasonable to carry out short trials with different amino acids because the response, or lack of it, usually indicates the underlying biochemical problem.

Treatment of this type should only be followed under the strict guidance of a qualified orthomolecular nutrition practitioner who is familiar with this type of orthomolecular psychiatry.

Most of the beneficial effects of tyrosine, or the side effects of an overdose, can be wiped out by the simultaneous administration of large amounts of neutral amino acids. Caffeine tends to lower plasma levels of tyrosine and could, therefore, increase the effects of stress in general.

Tryptophan and Depression

There are some types of depression that respond poorly or not at all to tyrosine and need tryptophan instead.

The clues to nontyrosine-dependent depressions are quite simple: sufferers will invariably crave sweets and consume carbohydrates (complex or otherwise) at every opportunity. Whenever they feel hungry—and this is usually midafternoon and late evenings—they will choose carbohydrates. They will often have gigantic sandwiches at ungodly hours—it is not the filling that is important, only the bread!

As a general rule, these depressed patients tend to have sleeping problems and usually respond well to tryptophan, another amino acid that crosses into the brain via the blood-brain barrier.

Tryptophan also comes from proteins, but, unlike tyrosine, it requires the simultaneous presence of carbohydrates in order to enter the brain.

Foods Containing Tryptophan

alfalfa	egg
baked beans	endive
beef	fennel
beet	fish
broccoli	milk
Brussels sprouts	nuts
carrot	soybeans
cauliflower	spinach
celery	sweet potato
chicken	turkey
chives	turnip
cottage cheese	watercress

Once it has entered the brain, tryptophan is then changed into sero-tonin, a neurotransmitter that can lift some types of depression, induce drowsiness, and stimulate immune functions.

Interestingly, the same combination of craving carbohydrates and experiencing depression can also be found in people suffering from bulimia and several types of premenstrual syndrome. Many cases of premenstrual syndrome respond well to oral supplements of tryptophan.

It is also interesting that most antidepressants cause people to gain weight, and scientists have been searching for a drug that does not cause this side effect. The latest one available is fluoxetine, and guess what—it exerts its antidepressant effect by artificially increasing brain levels of serotonin, the product of tryptophan.

THE CASE OF PAMELA X

Pamela was suffering from premenstrual tension (PMT) and depression during her period. After interviewing her, I decided her premenstrual syndrome was caused predominantly not by tension but by a combination of high levels of estrogen and depression. She was also overweight and craved sweets, especially before her periods.

Pamela found it difficult to fall asleep, yet she needed a lot of sleep in order to function at work, something she found herself less and less capable of doing. Her libido was all but gone, and her husband's flowers and dinners were doing nothing to encourage a sexual spark.

I prescribed a B-complex formula, plenty of oil of evening primrose, a teaspoon of honey, and tryptophan in tablet form to be taken at bedtime on an empty stomach. I also gave her magnesium to be taken daily starting halfway through her menstrual cycle, regular doses of vitamin E, and calcium.

Three months later Pamela's depression had ceased; she had lost weight, and her libido had returned.

Sunlight and Depression

The science that deals with our biological clocks and rhythms is called chronobiology. It is a growing area of research, and recent findings suggest that the actual timing of food intake, sleep patterns, and even the hour at which drugs are administered may be a great deal more important than we previously thought.

I am sure most of you know that we are supposed to experience a lift in moods in spring. It is the time of the year when our hormones are supposed to get up and get going and drive us to mate and engage in other hedonistic lapses of good sense.

This notion, buried deeply in folklore, actually has a lot of truth in it. As the days get longer, wildflowers poke their heads above the ground, the winter blues vanish, and new bursts of energy seem available on demand. This often happens to people who spend almost all the winter months in a state of mental hibernation—a sort of mind slush that slows them down and makes them feel depressed.

We now know that many people who suffer the blues all winter and then obtain a reprieve every spring suffer from seasonal affective disorder syndrome (SADS). The cause of their problems and their yearly spontaneous recovery are linked to their pineal gland.

Named because of its shape—it resembles a pine cone—the pineal gland is now recognized as the seat of our biological clock. Smaller than an aspirin tablet, it is the organ responsible for a human's daily rhythms, most animals' mating seasons, and also the daily and seasonal changes in biochemical functions.

The pineal gland is a "neuroendocrinal transducer," which means it translates input signals, such as light, into nerve impulses that in turn stimulate endocrine glands to produce a veritable cascade of hormones. These hormones control, affect, and modify almost all aspects of animal physiology, biochemistry, and behavior. When light signals are scarce or absent, the pineal gland activates two of its resident enzymes: N-acetyl transferase (NAT) and hydroxyindole-O-methyl-transferase (HIOMT). These enzymes then begin to turn serotonin into the hormone melatonin.

If you are susceptible, and SADS sufferers obviously are, the resulting lack of serotonin makes you depressed. With the coming of spring and more daylight, the process is reversed, and there is a lift in mood.

The Pineal Gland and Nature

Nearly all reptiles, amphibians, birds, fish, and mammals have a pineal gland, and the few that do not have cells that perform the same functions.

The pineal gland has been part of the animal world for at least 500 million years. Organs as ancient and widespread as the pineal gland are not there for the evolutionary ride alone; the importance of the functions of this little gland can be gathered by observing that when it is surgically removed the physiology and behavior of any animal is profoundly altered. Breeding cycles go haywire or stop altogether. Fish lose their protective colorings, making them easy victims of predators. Frogs and squirrels are no longer able to adjust their body temperature, and birds lose the desire to migrate. Even deer are affected by growing antlers at the wrong time. The pineal gland seems to adjust the whole physiology of animals to their environment.

Daylight and sunshine cause the pineal gland to make *less* melatonin from serotonin via N-acetyl transferase (NAT) and hydroxyindole-O-methyltransferase (HIOMT). As a result of this, more serotonin is available to help curb appetite in general and carbohydrates or sweets in particular. One sleeps better and tends to be less depressed.

In spite of all the important functions the pineal gland performs, it is not the master at all, as once believed. It is, in fact, a slave under the control of yet another "master clock": the suprachiasmatic nuclei (SCN). This mass of specialized brain cells controls the pineal gland's nightly output of NAT.

During winter, many animals hibernate and any mating urges cease. It is now believed that the hibernation process is triggered by melatonin and, as we have seen, the brain uses serotonin to make melatonin.

As daylight hours become shorter, the pineal produces more melatonin, and the incidence of SADS increases. Apart from being a good reason for extending daylight saving, it is interesting to note that increased serotonin plays a role in stimulating the immune system.

Have you ever noticed that when you are ill, especially when you have a viral infection such as the flu, you tend to sleep a lot? The body knows your immune system needs a little boosting and makes you sleepy by increasing serotonin levels. In turn, sleeping makes you conserve your energy, and so the cycle continues.

Knowing that sunshine decreases melatonin and, therefore, increases serotonin levels in the brain may help to explain why excessive sunbathing can make you so sleepy, while a brisk walk on a clear day can make you feel more alert.

SUNLIGHT VERSUS ARTIFICIAL LIGHT

Millions of people, especially in colder climates, spend a great part of their daily lives under some form of artificial light. Light bulbs emit light that differs greatly from sunshine. Sunlight casts a full range of colors as well as ultraviolet and infrared light. Incandescent light bulbs emit only the yellow, orange, and red portions of the spectrum.

Fluorescent lights work by passing a current through a tube filled with argon gas and mercury vapor. Fluorescent lights can be made to give off any combination of colors; however, early developers decided to use the yellow and green portions of the spectrum because the human eye is most sensitive to them. This gives the characteristic "cool-white" light with which we are all familiar.

Photobiologists are now finding that spending a lot of time exposed to only "cool-white" portions of the light spectrum can upset the delicate human biochemistry by altering the ratio of hormones. It can also cause calcium malabsorption and deficiencies as well as a need for additional vitamin A. Unshielded fluorescent light may also add ultraviolet radiation and cause sensitive people to become more susceptible to skin cancer.

To produce the required effects of natural light, full-spectrum light should be used.

THE CASE OF JOHN X

John was referred to me by one of my former students. "John is clearly suffering from hypoglycemia," I was told over the phone. "If he goes for as little as four hours without a meal he suffers headaches and brain fog and becomes extremely moody. Yet when I asked him to avoid refined carbohydrates and increase protein intake, he became very tired and depressed. I changed his diet to include more complex carbohydrates, and he improved somewhat but gained weight. He then had to go to Tasmania on business for a few weeks (in the middle of winter), and by the time he got back he was suicidal!"

John explained to me that as soon as he got to Hobart he became almost frantic about finding some ice cream. Unless he had some sweets, he would become terribly depressed. His job kept him indoors almost all day, and when he got to his hotel at night, he spent several hours working under artificial light.

John was suffering from SADS. I prescribed supplemental tryptophan, calcium, vitamin A, and vitamin B_3 and suggested that he spend at least a couple of hours each day walking around in the open air. I also explained to him that he should not spend too much time under fluorescent lighting and should attempt to change his home and office lights to the full-spectrum variety.

After a few weeks John had found his depression begin to lift. He told me that, as long as he continued to take care of his blood sugar he felt emotionally well.

Chemicals and Depression

Ask anyone what they think are the causes of depression, and you will hear many similar answers: lack of money, overwork, unhappy relationships, stress—the list goes on. Ask a professional with a general knowledge of science and medicine, and the list will be similar, however, with extra things such as hereditary factors, brain malfunctions, or severe illness. Doctors or psychiatrists will add various neurotransmitter imbalances, childhood traumas, and several diseases to that list.

If, however, you were to talk to an experienced environmental medicine practitioner or to an orthomolecular psychiatrist, you would learn that depression can also be caused by allergies or intolerances to a variety of foods, inhalants, and chemicals; or nutritional imbalances or deficiencies of vitamins, minerals, and amino acids. There is also a variety of seemingly unrelated conditions, such as candida infections, irritable bowel syndrome, and postviral syndrome, that can cause depression. Long-term low-grade exposure to toxic and foreign chemicals (xenobiotics) can also cause depression, whether you are allergic to them or not. (Naturally, the same applies to short-term overexposure.)

PROFOUND SENSITIVITY SYNDROME

While we all meet people who are emotionally very sensitive (those who cry at the drop of a hat), there appears to be a certain proportion of the population who are profoundly sensitive to a vast array of factors in their environment. This problem is called profound sensitivity syndrome (PSS). People suffering from PSS are usually creative, artistic, highly perceptive, and emotionally sensitive.

Some believe that people with PSS are more likely to suffer from autoimmune diseases such as lupus, multiple sclerosis, and arthritis. Because PSS sufferers perceive many events as stressful that others would consider trivial, they often suffer the physical consequences of chronic low-grade stress.

Environmental doctors have added a new dimension to this proposition. They argue, convincingly in my opinion and clinical experience, that people who are inherently emotionally hypersensitive are more likely to be susceptible to environmental pollutants and xenobiotics. Often, in fact, neuropsychiatric symptoms, such as depression, anxiety, and paranoia are the first noted manifestations of some physical illness.

Hereditary factors, past illness, or lifestyle can make some people's nervous system more susceptible to viral or chemical agents. Usually, such damage manifests itself as mood swings, agitation, feeling "spaced out," poor concentration, and memory impairment. All these are signs of central nervous system depression.

Environmental illness specialists also believe that chemical sensitivity can be transmitted from mother to child. Dr. William Rae, founder and director of the Environmental Health Center in Dallas, Texas, says:

> You can pass down chemicals and sensitivities from mother to child. It's seen in dope addicts and their babies, cigarette smokers and their babies, and alcoholics and their babies. So it's not really startling that other chemicals are passed down. It's the logical extension. The data is there. If the mother had ten parts of styrene (a highly toxic xenobiotic compound which some plastic coffee cups and some insulation materials are made of) in her blood, the child may have two, or three parts in his.

As a result of a parent's sensitivity, a child may be born with a predisposition toward profound sensitivity. Dr. Rae explains that conventional doctors and psychiatrists do not understand the interactions between the environment and human beings.

In his experience, a third of his depressed patients are so because they have been exposed to chloroform. He has tested thousands of depressed patients and, in many cases, found high levels of chloroform in their blood. Chloroform is an anesthetic and is in the steamy vapors that arise from the chlorine in our water during a long, hot shower. Now you know why a hot shower can be so relaxing and sleep-inducing, while a cold one tends to be invigorating.

What a lot of people do not know is that many solvents, such as trichloroethane, which is used in dry cleaning and many other industrial cleaning applications, can also affect your mental state and cause mood swings, depression, and even anxiety.

Another little-known fact is that many of these chemicals are partial alcohols and act like a central nervous system depressant. Because air pollution can contain staggering amounts (100 tons per year in the air of Dallas alone) of such xenobiotics, and because our detoxification pathways (mainly via the liver) are already very busy taking care of alcohol and many other xenobiotics, it is hardly surprising that depression is common.

Another xenobiotic that can precipitate depression, as well as other symptoms, is formaldehyde. It can affect the nervous system of profoundly sensitive people, causing depression, poor concentration, memory problems, and agitation.

How can we get such chemicals into our blood? Consider the following: if you place a lemon on a table a meter away, chances are you will be able to smell its fragrance. The reason is that the lemon, like everything else, decomposes ever so slightly, so that minute particles are inhaled—hence you can smell it.

Anything that can be smelled eventually enters your bloodstream. This process is known as outgassing. So if your new carpet, plastic fabric, or furniture outgasses, chances are some formaldehyde enters your blood. If you are profoundly sensitive, it can cause depression.

Depression and other emotional problems can also be caused by old viruses—viruses that were contracted years, even decades, before without them causing symptoms at the time. When such viruses are reactivated, mood swings and emotional problems can occur. This is also caused by postviral syndrome.

Fatigue, Depression, and Adrenal Exhaustion

Poor adrenal functions, excessively low cholesterol levels, and a lack of salt are often overlooked as a possible cause of depression and tiredness.

When the adrenals do not work as well as they should, the condition is known as chronic adrenal insufficiency, burnout syndrome, hypoadrenia, or hypoadrenocorticism.

It is not uncommon to find symptoms such as low blood pressure, hypoglycemia, impaired liver function, and salt cravings in people who have impaired or insufficient adrenal functions.

The adrenal glands consist of two parts: an outer, tough exterior called the cortex and an interior part called the medulla. The medulla produces the hormone called adrenaline. The adrenal medulla and the cortex are both under the control of the pituitary gland, which sits at the base of the brain and is itself controlled by the hypothalamus.

The hypothalamus is a tiny pocket, or ventricle, in the brain that acts like a bugging device on all incoming messages about sight, sound, taste, and smell. It translates these messages into chemical substances called releasing factors, and the releasing factors cause the pituitary gland to give off appropriate hormones, some of which affect the adrenal glands.

HYPOGLYCEMIA

When the body is under stress, the adrenal glands secrete glucocorticoids, which result in an increase in blood-sugar levels. The pancreas has to secrete insulin to cope with the increased blood sugar, and levels return to normal.

If, however, this happens too often, then both the adrenals and the pancreas are forced to work overtime. The pancreas may also overreact in these situations, causing blood-sugar levels to be constantly low. Low blood sugar is one possible cause for chronic fatigue.

It also stands to reason that if one's adrenals are working below par—as is often the case when one has been under stress for a long time—tiredness will be one of the inevitable results.

SALT

Another consequence of exhausted adrenals and many acute illnesses is that blood levels of sodium decrease.

The adrenals, which are in charge of this department, too, excrete special hormones called mineralocorticoids to help the body retain whatever salt it gets from the diet. If we eat too much salt, the result can be fluid retention and other complications; if there is not enough salt in the food we eat, the adrenals have to work much harder, and their efficiency suffers further.

Most doctors and many nutritionists believe that we already have too much salt in our diet. Yet many seem unaware that the connection between dietary salt and high blood pressure is not only far from proven, but that there is much scientific evidence showing that only a small percentage of people, specifically those sensitive to sodium, will have their blood pressure increased by dietary salt intake.

While attention is given to high blood pressure and risks of cardio-vascular disease, very little publicity is given to the very common condition of low blood pressure, which can make people tired, unable to concentrate, dizzy, and overweight. Generally speaking, symptoms will worsen if salt intake is reduced, and sometimes, if salt intake is increased, it will help to alleviate symptoms.

The regulation of sodium depends largely on a healthy pair of adrenals. During mental or physical stress, adrenal activity changes markedly (see Chapter 6 on stress). For example, during the course of an infection, considerable demands are made upon the adrenal glands.

The amount of hormones stored in adrenal tissue is sufficient for only a few minutes in the absence of continual synthesis. For this reason, the rate of synthesis is extremely important to the rate of secretion.

Sodium deficiencies are among the most common endocrine disorders in clinical medicine. Failure to initiate salt-balance corrections may result in heart problems.

Sodium deficiencies make the body respond via the adrenals, whereby their outpourings cause blood vessels to constrict, resulting in poor oxygenation and reduced removal of waste products, such as lactic acid, from the blood. Lactic acid is what causes the muscular aches that sometimes follow exceptionally strenuous and prolonged muscular activity. An increase of lactate, the ionic form of lactic acid, can make muscles ache and cause anxiety in susceptible individuals.

Not surprisingly, excessive lactate is also a suspected cause of the muscular problems experienced by sufferers of chronic fatigue syndrome. In addition, many of the "nerve" problems associated with chronic fatigue syndrome, such as anxiety, fearfulness, tension, and irritability, can also be caused by excessive levels of lactate in the bloodstream. This type of anxiety is known as lactate-induced anxiety syndrome (LIAS) and is discussed in the chapter on mood swings. (See Chapter 2.)

CHOLESTEROL AND LIVER FUNCTIONS

Today many people endeavor to lower their cholesterol levels. Unfortunately, too little cholesterol can be just as bad as too much.

What most of us do not realize is that cholesterol performs several important functions. It is one of the ways in which the body disposes of some chemicals, notably mercury. Additionally, cholesterol is an important source of adrenal hormones. The adrenals are usually filled with cholesterol, which is transformed into adrenaline in the presence of vitamin C. If we run short of these hormones because of a shortage of cholesterol, adrenal insufficiency may occur, and such a sudden or excessive reduction in cholesterol may cause a lowering of blood pressure and swelling of the tissues with salt and water.

Cholesterol is manufactured and controlled by the liver. So when you are under stress, the body, in its wisdom, tells your liver to make more cholesterol. This ensures that the adrenals have enough to manufacture the extra stress hormones you need. This is one of the reasons why some people have increased levels of cholesterol when they are under stress, even though they may be following a low-cholesterol diet.

When we are exposed to foreign chemicals, an already bad situation is made worse because the liver has to work even harder to detoxify our system and to manufacture cholesterol. Many of the pathways used in the detoxification process are shared by alcohol and chemicals for which the liver is responsible.

MUSCULAR WEAKNESS AND ACHES

Many people who suffer with chronic fatigue also have problems with muscular weakness and aches. The adrenal cortex has a powerful and direct influence on muscle responses.

If we look at Addison's disease, the classic disease involving impaired adrenal functions, we see that among its symptoms are poor concentration, poor memory, drowsiness, depression, insomnia, restlessness, apprehension or anxiety, irritability, headaches, temporary blurring of vision, dizziness, and tinnitus (ringing in the ears).

All those symptoms are also common in most people who suffer with chronic and unexplained fatigue. This, of course, does not imply that if you are unusually tired, or even if you are more tired than usual, and somewhat depressed, that you are a victim of chronic fatigue syndrome or Addison's disease.

However, we must question the possibility that many chronic fatigue sufferers exhibit a degree of adrenal insufficiency. Perhaps then we may find a surprisingly high incidence of subclinical hypoadrenocorticism among them.

HOW TO IMPROVE ADRENAL FUNCTIONS

Worn-out adrenal glands can be helped by oral supplements of vitamin B_5 (also known as calcium pantothenate or pantothenic acid), which is found in eggs, wheat germ, licorice, salt, and a high-protein diet that is not excessively low in cholesterol.

Foods High in Vitamin B_5 (Pantothenic Acid)

avocado	lobster
bean sprouts	mackerel
beef	mushrooms
chicken	peanuts
clams	pineapple
crab	salmon
egg	sardines
haddock	soybeans
lentils	watermelon
liver (beef, pork)	wheat germ

Foods High in Vitamin C (Ascorbic Acid)

alfalfa	citrus fruit (lemons, oranges)
banana	guava
berries (blueberries,	kidney
gooseberries rasp-	liver (beef)
berries, strawberries)	oysters

Vitamin C plays an important role not only in maintaining the adrenals' integrity but also in helping the conversion of cholesterol to adrenal hormones.

Other important nutrients are vitamin A, vitamin B_2 (riboflavin), zinc, magnesium, and the amino acid tyrosine, which requires both vitamin C and calcium for its utilization.

Korean ginseng and herbs such as safflower, parsley, sarsaparilla, kelp, sage, and savory also tend to help adrenal functions. A daily dose of garlic and sesame butter is also beneficial.

Note that licorice is inadvisable in cases of high blood pressure, potassium deficiency, and kidney disease. It also has a laxative effect.

Brazil nuts	potato
broccoli	spinach
Brussels sprouts	sweet potato
cabbage	tomatoes
cantaloupe	vegetables (green leafy ones)
cauliflower	watermelon
peppers (green, red)	

Foods High in Vitamin A

butter	milk
carrots	oysters
crab	salmon
cream cheese	spinach
egg	squash
grapefruit	sweet potato
halibut	swordfish
liver (beef, fish)	tomato
margarine	vegetables (dark green,
melons	leafy ones)

Foods High in Zinc

beef	milk
bran	mushrooms
Brazil nuts	oatmeal
brown rice	oysters
crab	pork
egg	pumpkin seeds
grains	sunflower seeds
herring	tuna
kidney	veal
lamb	yeast (brewer's)

Foods High in Magnesium

almonds	lima beans
apricots, dried	molasses
avocado	oatmeal
baked beans	peaches
barley	peanuts
beef	peas
Brazil nuts	pecans
carrots (raw)	pork
cashews	potato
chicken	rice
citrus fruits	sesame
corn	soybeans
crab	tomato (raw)
dates	vegetables (dark green leafy ones)
fish (flounder, salmon, tuna)	wheat germ
lentils	

Korean ginseng is also contraindicated in some cases of female hormonal and gynecological problems, such as menorrhagia (abnormal bleeding from the uterus).

Tyrosine can aggravate some psychiatric disorders and is contraindicated in cases of melanoma cancer and in immune dysfunctions where the natural killer cells (NK) are low.

HOW TO ASSESS ADRENAL INSUFFICIENCY

One of the simplest ways to assess the possibility of adrenal insufficiency is to measure the blood pressure while the patient has been sitting or lying down in a comfortable position for a few minutes and again immediately after the patient has quickly moved to a standing position.

The systolic pressure should be higher when the patient stands up suddenly. If it fails to increase or, worse still, if it decreases, then it indicates the possibility of adrenal impairment. The degree by which systolic blood pressure drops when in the standing position gives the therapist a rough estimate as to the degree of adrenal insufficiency.

A more elaborate method is the "water loading" test. This can be carried out at home with simple instructions from a therapist, who should then interpret the results. This test is contraindicated in people with known kidney diseases.

Foods High in Vitamin B$_2$ (Riboflavin)

almonds	flour
beans	mackerel
beef (kidney, heart, liver)	milk
black currants	mushrooms
Brazil nuts	oysters
cheese	perch
chicken (liver)	rice
clams	salmon
cod	spinach
collard	trout
egg	

AGING AND ALZHEIMER'S DISEASE

W̶e begin to die the day we are born" is a rather unpalatable truism; however, growing old does not necessarily mean becoming senile. In fact, senility may well be somewhat of a myth, according to some scientists who study the aging process.

Until recently, symptoms such as memory loss, difficulties with bowel control, getting dressed, and driving a car were considered a natural consequence of aging. Today, this view has been discarded by the scientific community. Even at 80, a decline in mental capacity is thought of as a disease, not a natural occurrence.

As we increase our life span, afflictions that were once rare are now becoming common. As the century draws to a close, we face the unprecedented situation in which as many as 30 percent of citizens of most advanced countries may be geriatrics.

Leading Australian expert Dr. Henry Brodaty of Prince Henry Hospital, Sydney, claims that senile dementia is 14 times more common than multiple sclerosis, and while it generally attacks older people, it can sometimes strike people in their forties. (The youngest case known was that of a six-year-old girl.) By the year 2000, it is estimated that 10 percent of those over 65 may suffer with senile dementia.

Alzheimer's Disease

Alzheimer's disease has been called "the quiet epidemic," "the silent disease," and "the funeral that never ends." But whatever the name, the disastrous effects it has on its victims have been aptly described as a total destruction of the individual.

Senile dementia is the overall term given to many different diseases producing dementia. Over 50 percent of dementia cases are considered to be sufferers of Alzheimer's disease. More than 1.5 million Americans now have Alzheimer's disease. It is estimated that by the year 2000 there will be 2 million.

The disease was first identified in 1906 by the German physician Alois Alzheimer. After the death of one of his patients, a 51-year-old woman with severe memory loss and mental confusion, Dr. Alzheimer decided to conduct an autopsy on her brain. He found the two distinctive characteristics of the disease: tangled lumps of brain nerve fibers and pockets of disintegrated nerve-cell branches.

There is a popular misconception that Alzheimer's disease can be readily diagnosed by its symptoms. However, diagnosis while the patient is still alive remains largely a process of elimination. If, after a battery of tests, a physician can exclude multiple brain infarcts (a series of small strokes within the brain), Parkinson's disease, alcoholism, arteriosclerosis of the brain, tumors, depression, adverse drug reactions and side effects, and psychiatric problems (all possible causes of dementia), then the diagnosis is made by default. The only way to be absolutely certain if someone suffered from Alzheimer's disease is to examine the brain after death.

The structural changes in the brain can be clearly seen with a low-powered microscope and seem to be concentrated in the cerebral cortex (where thought processes originate) and the hippocampus (which plays a special role in learning and memory processes).

The disease would be easier to detect and treat if we knew exactly what causes it.

Another popular misconception about Alzheimer's disease is that certain signs, such as loss of memory, are the only, or at least the only sure, indications of the disease. Unfortunately, both the onset and progress of Alzheimer's disease are so insidious that they often escape recognition for months and even years. In addition, the early symptoms are varied and not easy to detect.

Consider the following. A woman cannot remember whether she turned off the stove or locked the front door. A son noticed that his mother was not able to balance her checkbook and count change at the local grocery store. A businessman notices that his wife uncharacteristically starts to indulge in wild spending sprees and is unable to make sense of simple phone messages. The wife of a handyman noticed a deterioration in her husband's quality of workmanship because walls were unevenly painted and a set of wall cabinets was so crooked the doors would not shut properly. Such aberrations are the marks that often signal the onset of Alzheimer's disease.

Is aluminum a cause of Alzheimer's disease? Are low levels of certain neurotransmitters the result of a systems failure, which then produces the disease, or does Alzheimer's disease cause such failures and/or low levels of brain chemicals? Could the fault lie in altered patterns of receptors, which then fail to respond adequately to neurotransmitters? Is it that a deficiency of some essential metal, such as calcium, magnesium, or manganese, is suspected of allowing aluminum and perhaps other brain toxins to accumulate in the brain?

Stages of Alzheimer's Disease

Age: abilities acquired	Disease stage: abilities lost
15+: get and hold a job	*Borderline*: hold job
7–12: handle money	*Early stages*: simple finances
5–7: select proper clothes	*Early stages*: select clothes
5: put on clothes	*Moderate stage*: put on clothes
4: go to toilet alone	*Severe*: go to toilet alone
4: shower unaided	*Severe*: shower unaided
3–4: control bladder	*Late*: control bladder
2–3: control bowels	*Late*: just control bowels
15 *months*: speak a few words	*Late*: just speak a few words
1 *year*: speak one word	*Late*: speak one word
1 *year*: walk	*Late*: walk
6–9 *months*: sit up unaided	*Late*: barely sit up unaided
2–3 *months*: smile	*Late*: smile

Or are there other factors, such as viral diseases, which disrupt natural protective mechanisms and allow the passage of toxic metals into the brain across the blood-brain barrier? Let us look at some of the current theories, hypotheses, and ideas about Alzheimer's disease.

HEREDITY

Heredity may play a role because Alzheimer's disease often occurs in members of the same family. A sibling of an Alzheimer's disease sufferer has a 50 percent chance of developing the disease if that person lives long enough for the symptoms to manifest themselves. Perhaps its onset is influenced or triggered by several genes so that anyone carrying them would become a sufferer only if they all combined simultaneously.

Apart from the statistical evidence, some scientists believe that because almost all Down's syndrome sufferers develop Alzheimer's disease by the age of 40, there is a strong heredity factor. So strongly do some medical scientists believe in this theory that at least one Australian doctor claims he has found a way with nutritional therapy to prevent Alzheimer's disease and in some cases even reverse some of its effects.

Dr. Chris Reading, a Sydney psychiatrist who is widely recognized as Australia's pioneer of nutritional psychiatry, is also an expert in human genetics and believes he has found a link between illnesses such as leukemia, Alzheimer's disease, Down's syndrome, and schizophrenia. "These diseases often occur over several generations of the same family and appear to have similar causes," says Dr. Reading.

Dr. Reading's success with sufferers of Alzheimer's disease stems from his work with Down's syndrome children. After testing 4,000 patients over a six-year period, he discovered that some vitamin and mineral deficiencies as well as inherited food or chemical allergies or intolerances cause abnormal growths, and the development of Alzheimer's disease in children with Down's syndrome.

If their nutritional problems and allergies are treated in time, there is a strong likelihood that they will not develop Alzheimer's disease in later years. Dr. Reading is currently working to assess if such preventive measures may apply to other susceptible individuals and perhaps to the general population.

VIRUSES

Knowing that many Alzheimer's disease sufferers seldom appear ill and hardly ever show signs of infection, such as a fever or elevated white cell count, it seems strange that anyone should consider viral infections as a possible cause.

However, some scientists speculate that one of the slow viruses may be responsible. Since the discovery in the 1960s of viruses that are capable of causing harm years after the original infection has taken place, we have come to realize that it is possible a viral agent may cause Alzheimer's disease and perhaps several other diseases that currently have no explanation.

The possibility exists that a virus may impair the activity or synthesis of key brain enzymes or even neurotransmitters.

ABNORMAL PROTEINS

There is little doubt that Alzheimer's disease is associated with protein abnormalities. The nerve cells tangle, and complex proteins (amyloids) surround and invade both cerebral blood vessels and degenerating nerve endings.

These are characteristic findings in Alzheimer's disease, but so far nobody has been able to say if they are the cause or the effect of the disease. Indeed, the possibility exists that, if they are abnormal, the synthesis of the proteins could be dictated by abnormal genes, making it hereditary or a genetic abnormality.

It may also be possible that abnormal or defective enzymes are activated by environmental toxins and then synthesize modified proteins, which essentially choke normal brain cells. These protein bundles, called neurofibrillary tangles, are numerous in the brain stem neurons, which release neurotransmitters in general and acetylcholine in particular.

The amyloids tend to collect in the middle layers of blood vessels in the brain and advance outward, where they eventually weaken and even replace the walls. This weakening of the blood-vessel walls may explain the local hemorrhages, which are common in the last stages of Alzheimer's disease.

Local hemorrhages are technically known as strokes. Repeated small cerebral strokes can give rise to the same symptoms as someone suffering late stage Alzheimer's disease. It is often difficult to know until after death if the patient is suffering from true Alzheimer's disease.

NEUROTRANSMITTERS

Neurotransmitters are natural chemicals that the brain makes from common amino acids that enable brain cells to communicate with each other; they are the basic constituents of proteins derived from the food we eat every day. In other words, they are chemical messengers within the brain and central nervous system.

While each neurotransmitter has a specific function in the brain, most have more than one, and in almost all cases, the quantity of each is not always as important as the ratio between two or more of them at any time. Even if one believes that Alzheimer's disease needs a combination of factors to occur, the fact remains that one or more neurotransmitters are linked with the disease.

In the mid-1970s Dr. Peter Davies, then at the Institute of Neurology in London, showed that the brains of people with Alzheimer's disease contained drastically reduced levels (up to 90 percent) of a key enzyme, choline acetyltransferase (CAT). This enzyme is needed by the brain to produce a chemical neurotransmitter known as acetylcholine, which is made from the amino acid choline and acetyl coenzyme A (requiring vitamin B_1 and vitamin B_5).

When David Drachman of the University of Massachusetts Medical Center administered a drug called Scopolamine (known to interfere with acetylcholine memory mechanisms), the temporary state of mental confusion and memory loss was virtually indistinguishable from that of someone with Alzheimer's disease. This supports the theory that memory impairment is associated with a decrease in acetylcholine levels.

Experiments calculated to increase levels of CAT enzymes or to reduce the rate of acetylcholine breakdown show that the rate at which the neurotransmitter is synthesized is limited not necessarily by the amount of enzymes but by the availability of the precursor substances from which acetylcholine is manufactured—choline and acetyl coenzyme A.

Foods High in Choline

bean sprouts	liver (beef, pork)
beef	milk
egg yolk	peanuts
garbanzo beans	split peas
green beans	soy
lentils	

Giving patients large amounts of supplemental choline or lecithin has been shown to help to reduce the symptoms of Alzheimer's disease. A carefully controlled study by Raymond Levy of the University of London Faculty of Medicine found continuing behavioral improvements in eight out of 24 patients treated in this way. While this is encouraging, results such as these strongly suggest that there are several forms of Alzheimer's disease.

Because autopsies of Alzheimer's disease sufferers reveal physical destruction of nerve cell terminals, it is also possible that, when faced with a shortage of choline, which is needed to synthesize acetylcholine, the brain cannibalizes some of its own cell membranes for their content of phosphatidlycholine, a ready source of choline.

The neurotransmitter hypothesis does not preclude environmental toxins or nutrient deficiencies (other than choline, vitamin B_1, and vitamin B_5) from being causes of Alzheimer's disease, because toxins such as aluminum may well block neurotransmitters, their synthesis, or perhaps their activity. The complex interactions of nutrients, such as vitamins and minerals, also make it possible that a specific deficiency of one of these may upset the delicate balance between neurotransmitters, their precursors, or the enzymes necessary for their synthesis.

ENVIRONMENTAL DEFICIENCIES

Many people like to blame our deteriorating environment, particularly the chemicalization of air, water, and food supplies, for almost all our health problems. Others are convinced that deficiencies of various nutrients, especially vitamins and minerals, are at the root of all modern diseases.

However, these two factors very often interact in ways that cause, or at least trigger, many illnesses. When an individual is susceptible, either because of an inherent trait or because of heredity, any factor may well precipitate Alzheimer's disease without being able to prove a direct cause-and-effect relationship.

We know, for example, that people who smoke more than one packet of cigarettes per day are four times more likely to get Alzheimer's disease than nonsmokers, yet no one is suggesting tobacco causes Alzheimer's disease. Many environmental factors exist which may trigger, aggravate, or cause Alzheimer's disease.

Consider the following. In the remote Pacific island of Guam, there is a tribe known as the Chamarros whose members suffer from a high incidence of amyotrophic lateral sclerosis (LAS), which causes progressive muscular wasting, Parkinson's disease-like tremors, Alzheimer's disease-like dementia, and neuron tangles. The Chamarros live in an area of Guam that is almost totally deficient in magnesium and calcium. We already know that a deficiency of calcium (or of vitamin D_3) tends to favor the accumulation of strontium 90, aluminum, and perhaps several other toxic metals.

Neuropathologist Dr. Daniel Perl of the University of Vermont College of Medicine in Colorado believes that the deficits of magnesium and calcium combined with the accumulation of heavy metals, such as aluminum, may play a role in the beginning of Alzheimer's disease.

Diuretics (water pills) are taken by millions of people in an effort to reduce high blood pressure and prevent heart disease. These drugs tend to increase the loss of several minerals such as calcium, magnesium, zinc and other essential micronutrients through the urinary system. Many people already have marginal levels of these nutrients and may not be left with enough to prevent toxic metals, such as aluminum, from accumulating in their brains.

Dr. Perl has also shown that the tangled nerve fibers in the brains of people suffering from Alzheimer's disease contain unusually large amounts of aluminum and that this metal, when injected into the brains of animals, leads to similar deterioration. His research suggests that aluminum accumulates preferentially in brain cells.

Other researchers, such as Donald Maclaughlin of the University of Toronto Faculty of Medicine, have shown that neuron tangles will develop in the brains of experimental animals when aluminum salts are injected.

Irreversible dementia is seen in some people who have undergone kidney dialyses with aluminum-rich solutions. In addition, we know that aluminum salts can inhibit some key brain enzymes as well as the transport of essential proteins (*Scientific American*, Jan. 1985, p. 48).

The possible involvement of aluminum in Alzheimer's disease was discussed widely at the Royal Society meeting in London (April 1987), and several scientists proposed that, quite apart from the obvious sources of this metal (see list on page 93), acid rain may be a major culprit. Aluminum is known to be the toxin responsible for the death of fish in streams and lakes rendered acidic by polluted rain. Aluminum dissolves in these waters instead of silicon; aluminum is toxic to humans, while silicon is essential for life.

Aluminum is the third most common element on earth, after oxygen and silicon, and the most prevalent metal in the crust of our planet. It is, therefore, not easy to avoid. Many commonly used items—antacids, deodorants, baking powders, and cookware—contain aluminum, but there are aluminum-free alternatives. To avoid aluminum in one's tap water or rainwater, the best solution seems to be using a good quality water filter.

There is still much debate as to whether the aluminum concentration is a cause or an effect of Alzheimer's disease. It is possible, however, that aluminum may cause the problem indirectly.

According to a study by Banks and Atkins of the Veterans Administration Medical Center and Department of Medicine at Tulane University School of Medicine in New Orleans, aluminum may alter the permeability of the natural barrier that protects the brain from unwanted substances: the blood-brain barrier (*The Lancet* 2 [1983]: 1227–1229).

It is speculated that this change in the permeability of the blood-brain barrier may allow other environmental toxins, and perhaps inimical

Common, and Not So Common, Sources of Aluminum

Aluminum cookware, including utensils

The following list outlines problems cooking in aluminum:

- Boiling water produces hydro-oxides, which are toxic.

- Boiling eggs produces phosphates, which inhibit the absorption of calcium.

- Boiling meat produces chlorides.

- Frying bacon increases nitrates.

- Vegetables tend to produce neutralizing factors that impede proper digestion of food.

- Teapots are particularly suspect because the tannic acid in tea tends to allow aluminum to leak into the beverage.

- Special chemicals called flocculating agents are used in water purification.

- Hot water pipes are sometimes made with cathodic corrosion preventatives made from aluminum.

Food additives

Aluminum is a common food additive in foods such as cheese, table salt, baking powders, pickles, maraschino cherries, vanilla powders, and bleached flours. Even milk formulas for babies contain up to 400 times more aluminum than that found in breast milk.

General additives

- toothpastes

- nasal sprays

- anti-perspirants

- dental fillings

- cigarette filters

- aspirin compounds

- pesticides (which also end up as residue in some foodstuffs) proteins, to enter the brain and alter its functions. We already have a tentative model for this in the case of epilepsy, which can be triggered, if not caused, by excessive amounts of the otherwise harmless and even essential vitamin folic acid leaking into the brain of people prone to seizures.

Apart from the fact that aluminum is ubiquitous, there is the problem with absorption. This toxic metal can be readily absorbed into the body through the gastrointestinal tract (*New England Journal of Medicine* 17, no. 310: 107).

Not many Americans realize that the sale of aluminum cookware is prohibited in Germany, France, Switzerland, Belgium, Hungary, and Brazil.

ALCOHOL

According to Professor David Hawks, director of the Western Australian Alcohol and Drugs Authority, alcohol abuse has reached almost epidemic proportions in Australia. However, there is a conspiracy of silence among the various authorities to suppress a number of reports that show that if the sum total of harm associated with alcohol was added up, the ill effects of all other drugs combined, including heroin and cocaine, would pale into insignificance.

To what extent long-term drinking affects the brain and how many cases of senility and Alzheimer's disease are, in fact, the result of the adverse effects of alcohol is anyone's guess. More than 10 million Americans are affected by alcohol abuse.

Alcohol exerts a powerful influence on the human brain. It stimulates the production of brain chemicals called endorphins, which act as an anesthetic. Alcohol dulls physical pain and also depresses areas of the brain responsible for controlling behavior and coordination. In addition, it irritates the gut linings and can be responsible for malabsorption of nutrients essential for brain functions.

After all, almost without exception, every neurotransmitter used by the brain is made from a food-derived amino acid, and its synthesis requires the presence and coordination of several vitamins, minerals, and other essential nutrients.

This is evident from the fact that many neurological disorders are caused directly by a deficiency of vitamin B_1 (thiamine), which can

Foods High in Vitamin B₁ (Thiamine)

beef (heart, liver, kidney)	pork (liver)
Brazil nuts	poultry
cereals	pumpkin
fish (mackerel, perch,	soybeans
red snapper)	sunflower seeds
lamb	wheat
milk	wheat germ
oatmeal	yeast (brewer's)
peas and other legumes	

occur as a result of alcoholism. Professor Byron Kakulas, head of neuropathology at Royal Perth Hospital, claims that many of the negative effects of alcohol on the brain can be nullified by taking a few vitamins, especially vitamin B₁; doing so would immediately reduce some of the most common mental disorders associated with alcohol abuse. It should also be noted that vitamin B₁ is essential for one of the key biochemical steps in which acetylcholine (a brain neurotransmitter associated with Alzheimer's disease) is synthesized from the amino acid choline.

BLOOD SUGAR

We have become so involved with the problems of hypoglycemia (low or fluctuating blood sugar) that we tend to forget some of the devastating effects that high blood-sugar (glucose) levels can cause.

We have long known that diabetics tend to be prone to infections and that their susceptibility is influenced by how well the disease (or blood-sugar level) is controlled. We also know that several of the complications of diabetes, including senile cataracts, joint stiffness, and atherosclerosis, mimic the degenerative processes of old age.

Collagen, the most abundant extracellular protein that glues cells together, degenerates when it is exposed to glucose. This means that blood sugar may play a role in the tissue changes associated with degenerative processes such as aging. We do not know at this stage if these changes extend to, or are able to influence, brain cells, but it gives people another good reason not to eat excessive amounts of sweets.

You may think that this exonerates hypoglycemia (low blood sugar) as even a circumstantial culprit in Alzheimer's disease. Unfortunately, this is not so.

THE BLOOD FLOW–HYPOGLYCEMIA–HYPOXIA HYPOTHESIS

Chiropractors know only too well how many health problems can be relieved or cured by manipulations calculated to increase circulation in general and to specific areas. The normal blood flow to the brain tends to diminish by about 20 percent between the early 30s and 60s, but the brain compensates for this by extracting proportionally more oxygen from the blood.

In Alzheimer's disease, blood flow diminishes more than average, and the associated compensatory uptake of oxygen does not happen. Both the blood flow and oxygen consumption continue to decline equally in someone suffering from Alzheimer's disease.

Dr. Frank Benson of the University of California at Los Angeles School of Medicine found that as little as half the normal amounts of glucose were consumed by the brains of those with Alzheimer's disease. Glucose provides brain cells with all their energy requirements; however, this is only possible if oxygen is available at the same time.

Other researchers have found that levels of special enzymes needed to convert glucose to energy are deficient in brain samples of people affected by Alzheimer's disease. Can these factors be influenced by regular chiropractic treatment, exercise, good diet, and a healthy lifestyle?

Common sense would say so. As old age approaches, what can you do to avoid, or at least try to prevent, becoming a victim of Alzheimer's disease? Here are a few tips:

- Make sure your blood-sugar levels are normal and under control. A glucose tolerance test (GTT) is one way to be sure. If there is a history of diabetes in your family, then these checks should be done periodically. In general, though, it is advisable to avoid excessive sugars, sweets, and refined carbohydrates as well as alcohol.

- If you have the faintest suspicion that you are allergic or intolerant to anything, be it food, chemicals, or inhalants, have someone check this out and arrange prompt treatment.

- Avoid all additives, colorants, pesticides, toxic chemicals, and pollution sources.

- Unless absolutely necessary, do not use drugs or medicines that will negatively affect your blood flow, amino acid utilization or absorption, brain function, mineral and vitamin absorption, or metabolism. If you have to take some medicines, make sure you also take the appropriate vitamins, essential nutrients, and mineral supplements to compensate for this.

- Do all you can to avoid succumbing to viral infections. At the very least, this means taking daily supplements of a strong vitamin C plus zinc compound.

- Make sure your body is getting the best from foods you eat by ensuring that your digestive system is performing well. This may mean supplementary hydrochloric acid and biotin (especially if you are over 50) and digestive enzymes. Remember that some protein foods, such as eggs and fish, may actually enhance brain functions in old age.

- Take choline supplements (in lecithin form) and never go short of vitamin B_1 and vitamin B_5, especially if you drink alcohol or eat lots of sweets and refined carbohydrates.

- Make sure you get enough calcium, magnesium, and vitamin D_3, especially if you are exposed to aluminum.

- Avoid aluminum. Drink from glass containers and wrap your food in plain waxed paper.

- Use a good water filter.

- Drink moderate amounts of alcohol with meals only.

- Get plenty of exercise and fresh air to ensure good circulation.

- Vitamin E and niacin help blood flow, so take some every day.

- Have regular chiropractic or osteopathic adjustments to increase blood flow through your body and to your brain.

STRESS

CHAPTER 6

People everywhere suffer from stress. Doctors prescribe tranquilizers for it, politicians retire because of it, and mystics teach ways to try to overcome it.

However, as bad as we may think it is, stress is an essential process that keeps our adrenal glands working. When stress is too much though, a potentially dangerous situation arises. Our metabolism is unable to adjust, and this paves the way for various illnesses, degenerative diseases, and emotional problems.

Stress is activated by many factors, and in order to cope, we must be able to recognize the symptoms and have at our disposal a variety of resources to correct stress-induced imbalances.

What is Stress?

What is stress? Dr. Hans Selye, professor and director of the Institute of Experimental Medicine and Surgery at the University of Montreal, Canada, gives this definition in his book *Stress Without Distress* (Signet: New American Library, 1974):

> Everybody knows what stress is, and nobody knows what it is. The word stress, like success, failure or happiness, means different things to different people and, except for a few specialized scientists, no one has really tried to define it, although it has become part of our everyday vocabulary.

If the weather suddenly turns cold and windy, you are likely to shiver. If it gets hot, you'll sweat. If you eat too much sugar, your body will react by pumping out hormones that will cause the excess sugar to be stored or burned. Run uphill, and your heart will race faster. If you are in pain, if you are lonely, or if you lose too much blood from an injury, you experience stress.

While the mechanism of stress (the nonspecific response) is the same for all of us, the particular way in which each of us reacts to stress is different. In fact, one person may react in different ways to the same stress at different times. To paraphrase Hippocrates, "One man's stress is another man's ecstasy." Let's face it, some people do not mind physical pain, while others faint at the sight of blood.

Our ancestors lived precarious lives where each day was a stressful challenge just to find enough food to stay alive. Why, then, is stress more of a problem these days? The answer lies in the fact that primitive humans always took some physical action in response to stress and, in so doing, got it out of their system—they either killed the wild beasts or were killed by them. The physical action necessary to combat stress, the "fight or flight" response, burned up energy, cholesterol, and superfluous hormones, and after a while, things returned to normal.

People are subjected to many different stresses every day, but unlike our ancestors, there is nowhere to run or nothing to attack—you just sit feeling sick and fuming under the action of powerful hormones. Enough of these events, and sooner or later the body or the mind is unable to cope and breaks down. This is called psychosomatic or psychogenic illness.

However, it should also be remembered that there are different types of stress and that not all stress is bad for you. Take, for example, events such as getting married, concluding a business deal, or winning a competitive event; all these are forms of stress. If you avoided all stress, which is actually impossible, you might live a little longer, but you might also die of boredom!

How Does Stress Affect Your Body?

Dr. Selye defines stress as "the nonspecific response of the body to any demands made upon it." The key word here is nonspecific—the responses that cannot be seen. You can, however, see the obvious *spe-*

cific effects of some of the nonspecific responses, such as crying, fainting, shivering, sweating, and vomiting. All these are individual responses, which vary from time to time and person to person. Sometimes people *can* adjust to some stresses so that they no longer react to them in a particular way. You may break out in a cold sweat the first time you fly, but after a few times you adjust to it.

The nonspecific responses are those that are going on off camera—down in the engine room, so to speak. The nonspecific response causes the specific response in order to make the body adjust to the situation. If you get cold enough, you will shiver. Because shivering is motion, and motion creates heat, the body temperature rises. The body has adjusted.

In order to understand how the body adjusts to nonspecific responses, it helps to know something about the production of hormones secreted by the endocrine system. The adrenal glands sit on top of each kidney and produce the hormone adrenaline. Aggression, drive, and energy are what we associate with adrenaline. However, the adrenals are under the rule of a little gland that sits at the base of the skull, called the pituitary, and this gland is controlled by the hypothalamus.

The hypothalamus is a pocket, or ventricle, in the brain that acts as a monitoring device on all incoming messages from both outside and inside the body, including sound, taste, smell, blood pressure, acidity, and fluid concentrations in the blood. The hypothalamus is also called the neuroendrocrinal transducer because it translates (transduces) messages from nerve impulses into endocrinal (hormonal) messages.

These messages are translated into chemicals called releasing factors, hormone-like substances that travel to the pituitary and cause it to send off releasing hormones. The adrenals get some of these chemical messages (as well as others from the autonomic nervous system), and the alarm bell goes off!

Whether the alarm is caused by an enzyme in distress because we have eaten foods we cannot cope with or because we hear the baby crying, the adrenaline pours out into the bloodstream. Once this happens, the heart pumps faster, blood pressure rises, air passages enlarge, blood is drawn from the skin to muscles (now you know why your face becomes white with fear), and digestion is interrupted.

The blood, full of adrenaline, then reaches the pituitary and causes more hormones to shoot down to the other half of the adrenals, causing them to start pumping out some of their many hormones. Meantime, the thyroid, parathyroid, pancreas, and sex glands begin to secrete some of their particular hormones, too.

The result of this biochemical process is the body being revved up by little shock waves and prepared for action. However, too often nowadays, the strenuous action that makes use of all these functions does not follow.

Stress Concept of Disease

Dr. Selye put all the assorted miseries of the endocrine system into a neat package, which he called the "stress concept of disease."

During experiments in which he was injecting rats with different substances, he noticed that all the animals developed enlarged adrenal glands (a sure sign of overwork); their thymus, spleen, and lymph nodes shrank; and they developed ulcers.

Eventually, he discovered that practically all toxic substances, whether chemicals or drugs, could cause practically the same effects. Looking at humans, Dr. Selye found that these responses occurred in all kinds of patients, whether suffering from cancer, infections, or psychological stress.

If the mechanism is the same, why does stress affect different people in so many different ways, whereas the rats all got ulcers? Dr. Selye proposed that this was because animals used in experiments tend to be of the same breed, the same age, and even from the same litter, whereas humans have environmental differences, hereditary weakness, different occupational stresses, different emotional reactions, and a great difference in nutritional status.

It is a question of where the weak link is—that is, why tension at work will give one person high blood pressure, another an ulcer, and another a headache. Yet all these have one common factor: the alarm went off, and the endocrinal glands went to work pushing out their hormones.

Major substances released by the adrenals are the glucocorticoids, which increase blood-sugar levels so more energy is available. In response to this, the pancreas must then secrete insulin to bring blood-sugar levels down again when all the excitement is over. So even a candy bar or excess sugar can act as a form of stress.

Not only does the pancreas resent having to deal with an extra sudden rise in blood sugar, but if it happens too often, it may overreact so violently that blood-sugar levels fall too much. When this happens, the body has to create more blood sugar, often out of body proteins, or more sugar has to be eaten. As a result, the vicious circle starts all over again, and the body is then in the constant grip of biochemical stress. This last example is a form of hypoglycemia.

The adrenals also secrete cortisone, which dulls the body's immune response. You get a cold, flu, and other infections more easily when you are overstressed.

The thyroid is also affected by stress and tells the body to increase its metabolic rate. This means that fat stores are raided to make extra energy, body proteins are also sometimes broken down, calcium is leached from the bones, vitamins are used up more quickly, and the gastrointestinal tract races overtime, sometimes producing diarrhea. So when you are still huffing and puffing hours (even days) after the stressful event, the situation gets serious.

The effects of stress are cumulative. In other words, constant little stresses add up and can eventually produce greater health problems. Take noise, for example. It has been found that people living near airports or on flight paths tend to have more illnesses, especially cardiovascular illness, than those who do not. Even though you get used to the noise, the body's alarm bell still goes off every time a plane lands or takes off.

Over the years, the long-term effects of stress hormones pouring out at all hours of the day and night can produce disastrous results: immune responses are lowered, the kidneys and heart are overworked, blood pressure goes up, diabetes is more likely (because glucocorticoids tend to elevate blood-sugar levels), and the pancreas is hard-pressed to keep up the extra supply of insulin needed.

Stress and the Food You Eat

In our modern society, one of the most overworked organs is the liver. This is because, among other things, it has to keep changing the molecules of foods that we eat into different ones—some for storage, some for tissue building, and some for antibodies.

The liver also has to detoxify practically every foreign chemical we eat (antibiotics, colorings, preservatives), as well as excess fats, excess carbohydrates, excess proteins, and all alcohol. And if all this is not enough, it also has to break down many hormones after they have carried out messages.

If we continually pile up more and more work on the liver—as we do every time we take a drug, eat too much of something, drink too much, or inhale or ingest chemicals—its energy goes down. The liver then has less energy left to take care of stress hormones, and so they remain in the bloodstream longer than they should, and their negative side effects accumulate.

By eating overrefined, processed foods, we place our body under subtle but relentless stresses. While we are doing this, we are also depleting our stores of vitamins and other essential coworkers of our enzyme system. We place undue strain on the machinery of our body, and we become more and more susceptible to a whole range of diseases of the body and the mind.

There is no clear-cut cause-and-effect correlation between what we eat and getting cancer, bronchitis, or depression, but you may well find that air pollution, food additives, plus an inability to adapt to or cope with some unhealthy foods, plus the stresses of modern life, can all add up to illness. Everyone is biochemically unique: one man's meat can literally be another man's poison.

How to Avoid Stress By Diet

1. Find out whether you are unsuited to a certain type of diet. Vegetarianism is considered a healthy diet. However, if you happen to be affected by natural compounds found in many fruits and vegetables called salicylates, your choice of fruit and

vegetables will be very restricted. Most nutritionists are able to arrange for tests to assess the suitability of any given diet.

2. Once you have established a diet that agrees with your metabolism, determine which foods within that dietary regime cause your body less stress. For example, you may find out that you are sensitive to certain types of grains or that dairy foods cause you a problem, and so these should be avoided.

3. Try to avoid eating large amounts of refined and processed foods. If you are partial to certain foods that fall into this category, remember to give your body a break from these by eating fresh, simple foods.

4. Remember to supplement your diet with appropriate vitamins and minerals to help your enzymes function properly. Taking vitamins specific to your individual needs will also help your body to resist and withstand stress.

By following these simple steps you can avoid some of the everyday stresses that are placed on your body.

Strange, isn't it, that everybody knows that working too hard or sleeping too little are both stresses that should be avoided whenever possible, but fewer people are aware that refined, processed foods with preservatives and additives are just as much a source of subtle but continuous biochemical stress on your body.

Let us imagine that health and stress are the scales of justice. On one side you have "stress resistance" (50 grams) and on the other side you have "unavoidable stresses" (50 grams). If your "unavoidable stresses" are polluted air (ten grams), take-out foods (15 grams), and alcohol (ten grams), then you only have 15 grams left before you have tipped the scales beyond your stress resistance.

There are many people who seem to understand this credit and debit approach to health. It is not uncommon to find smokers who take more care of their diet and take special supplements to minimize the effects of smoking, or people who will eat dessert only if they have faithfully stuck to their exercise schedule.

These people are not fooling themselves, because little things do make a difference, and they have grasped the essential point: health is balance.

PREMENSTRUAL SYNDROME

CHAPTER 7

Until recently the best help that was offered for premenstrual syndrome was a tranquilizer, and more often than not, the unhappy sufferers were advised to take control of themselves. Today there is a veritable cornucopia of premenstrual tension remedies, mostly in the form of nutritional supplements or herbs. Some of these work for some women some of the time. There are, however, reasons why it is difficult to treat all sufferers successfully.

We are now discovering that there are many different types of premenstrual syndromes (which should not surprise anybody, considering that females are even more biochemically unique than males), which can be helped by different types and combinations of supplements and diets.

Recent research and the experience of clinical practice have shown that some of our patients will get better no matter what formula they take, while others will not. In many instances, I have noted that some of my patients actually get worse with certain types of supplements, especially those containing yeast, large amounts of folic acid, and iron. The same applies to diets: while most women benefit from avoiding fatty animal meats, some actually become worse if they switch to a complete vegetarian diet.

Premenstrual tension (PMT), as the syndrome is popularly referred to, can cause wild and uncontrollable mood swings, and in most cases, it is treatable provided the therapist can formulate a diet and supplements regimen suited to the individual.

Types of Premenstrual Syndrome

Specialists now divide premenstrual syndrome sufferers into five distinct subgroups. At the Complementary and Environmental Medicine Center in Sydney, we have successfully treated many thousands of patients with premenstrual syndrome and recognized at least seven subgroups with varying symptoms for which a combination of dietary and supplementary treatments may be useful.

A CASE OF PREMENSTRUAL BLUES AND OTHER PROBLEMS

Sally walked into my office looking like a picture of dejection: "I am 26 years old and for at least one week every month I feel like I'm 96! I become depressed, have incredible cravings for chocolate (which I binge on), and retain pounds of fluid. My skin gets ruined, and it takes weeks before it starts to look presentable again. By then, my next period is due, and the whole thing starts again!"

I asked Sally about her past pregnancies, and she told me that she had suffered with toxemia both times. When I heard this I explained to her that vitamin B_6 is reported to prevent and even cure toxemia during pregnancy. Interestingly, the same vitamin also has a reputation for reducing premenstrual depression, anxiety, and the flareup of skin conditions associated with estrogen sensitivities. It also exerts a diuretic effect and thus helps to reduce fluid retention.

I prescribed vitamin B_6 to be taken three times a day with meals. I also asked Sally to take vitamin E, because this nutrient is not only a useful antioxidant and circulation booster but also helps to counteract the effects of any excessive estrogen. In addition, I prescribed the oil of evening primrose, which reduces many of the stress symptoms associated with premenstrual syndrome, especially mood swings. It does not, however, have any effect on estrogen or fluid retention.

Sally protested, "How many pills do you want me to take? I'll be so full I won't need to eat!" I told her, however, that this was not all to be prescribed as there were two other aspects of her premenstrual syndrome that required special attention. She not only craved and binged on chocolate every month, causing her to have constipation and skin flareups, but she also suffered a considerable amount of pain with her period.

"There is a particular nutrient, actually an amino acid, called DL-phenylalanine (DLPA), which not only acts as a powerful yet natural painkiller but is also a good antidepressant and stops most people from craving chocolate. The reason is that chocolate contains a natural chemical, phenylethylalanine, which is converted to DLPA in the body. If you can find this nutrient in other foods, then the craving for chocolate would be satisfied without eating chocolate.

So it was natural for Sally to seek solace with chocolate. However, DLPA would do the same job without making her constipated or causing any worsening of her skin. I also added a vitamin C formula to her regimen because her urine test showed practically no vitamin C, and this nutrient is a powerful antioxidant and a natural antihistamine.

I saw Sally again five weeks later and she looked, and apparently felt, like a new woman. "I could not believe it," she exclaimed. "I hardly noticed my last period. It came on almost without any warning! My skin looks quite normal and I feel happy."

Symptoms of Premenstrual Syndrome

Psychological symptoms: irritability, nervous tension, anxiety, mood swings, aggressiveness, fatigue, inability to dream, lack of sex drive, depression, poor memory, inability to think clearly, mental confusion, and food cravings

Physical symptoms: abdominal swelling, general increase in weight and fluid retention, headaches, swelling and tenderness of breasts, muscular weakness, body aches and pains

1. PMS-T (TENSION)

Symptoms: nervous tension, irritability, anxiety, aggressiveness, anger, uncontrollable mood swings, palpitations, crying spells, tantrums, and low libido

While some of the symptoms may be associated with, and perhaps aggravated by, high estrogen levels and a relative deficiency of progesterone, the most common contributing factors in PMS-T are excessive alcohol consumption, decreased liver function, the use of oral contraceptives, excessive consumption of sugars and refined carbohydrates, and a stressful lifestyle.

These patients appear to benefit from an intake of calcium (in the orotate form), vitamin B_6, magnesium, zinc, ascorbic acid, and a diet that contains a reasonable amount of proteins. Spirulina seems to be ideal for these patients. Oil of evening primrose can also help, while vitamin B_3 (pantothenic acid) can make them worse.

PMS-T patients are ideal candidates for hypnotherapy, counseling, biofeedback, and other forms of relaxation-inducing, stress-lowering techniques.

We have also found that PMS-T sufferers tend to have elevated sensitivity to excess copper in their food or liquid intake. They often drink lots of tap water and use the hot water tap to make tea and coffee, which can cause additional copper consumption. In addition to advising them on safer drinking techniques, such as the use of a water filter, zinc and vitamin C supplements are particularly useful.

Premenstrual Syndrome and Aggression

It has been estimated that 90 percent of all aggressive behavior in women occurs around the time of their menstrual period, and nearly half of all crimes committed by females are perpetrated during menstruation or just before. More than half of the female population of reproductive age suffers from premenstrual syndrome.

2. PMS-E (ESTROGEN)

Symptoms: most of the symptoms of PMS-T, in addition to breast swelling and tenderness, clotty menstrual blood, and fluid retention

PMS-E sufferers are diagnosed differently from PMS-T because of the likelihood that this condition is caused or aggravated by excessive estrogen.

In many cases these women tend to have periodic food cravings, but not always for sweet substances. PMS-E women are often adversely affected by oral contraceptives (because of the estrogen content) and insufficient progesterone, a hormone that has been used with some success in the medical treatment of PMS.

Hypothyroidism goes hand in hand with increased estrogen levels, so each patient has to be carefully examined for low thyroid function.

Excessive estrogen levels are also associated with heart disease and some forms of cancer. Carleton Frederick, author of *Breast Cancer*, suggests that breast tenderness and swelling and fluid retention may be aggravated by too much folic acid and para-aminobenzoic acid (PABA). Folic acid increases the effects of estrogen, and PABA can exacerbate some of its effects.

Some women on a high-vegetable, low-protein diet appear to have menstrual problems that are reversed when their intake of vegetables, especially carrots, is decreased. Apart from the fact that many vegetables are high in folic acid, and this could presumably affect susceptible females, carrots and other vegetables contain estrogen-like substances.

Many plants, such as clover, lucerne, rye grasses, and soya, contain plant phenols or isoflavones, which are substances known as phyto-estrogens because they mimic the activity of the natural female hormone. Phyto-estrogens are also present in cow's milk and are more prevalent in skim milk than regular milk.

PMS-E women should be given ample amounts of vitamin B_6, magnesium, and zinc but not B-complex formulas (which contain large amounts of folic acid), para-aminobenzoic acid, calcium pantothenate, or calcium. Although vitamin C is recommended, care must be taken not to use calcium ascorbate formulas, as this may lower magnesium levels. PMS-E women usually tend to consume large amounts of dairy products.

Excessive brain serotonin (5HT) can often cause aggressiveness, irritability, and mood swings. Because estrogen may already contribute to an elevation of those neurotransmitters, formulas containing tryptophan should be taken with care. While vitamin B_3 (niacin or niacinamide) can be of some benefit, care must be taken against excesses in self-prescribing. A certain amount of carbohydrates, about 30 grams (or the equivalent of one banana), tends to facilitate the transfer of tryptophan across the blood-brain barrier, as can any insulin-elevating food, but this is dependent on the amounts of tryptophan contained in the remaining portion of the meal. Foods containing high proportions of tryptophan should not be taken with sweets.

The liver helps to rid the body of excess estrogen, so any food that decreases liver functions, such as hepatotoxic drugs, should be avoided or carefully monitored.

Insufficient amino acids, B-complex deficiencies, and anything but the most moderate intake of alcohol (one or two drinks per day with meals) can aggravate PMS-E, and all patients should be screened for a history of hepatitis and other liver diseases.

Vitamin B_{15} (pangamic acid) may be useful in such cases. Again, magnesium and vitamin E along with oil of evening primrose are invalu-

---

Estrogen and the California Desert Quail

Estrogen acts as a natural contraceptive, and the delicate balance required for this hormone can be seen by investigating the California desert quail.

When there is little rain, these birds appear to breed less. It seems that during a drought the seeds on which the quail feed produce additional estrogen. This acts as a contraceptive, and therefore the number of birds competing for the dwindling food supplies is reduced. When rain is abundant, the estrogen content of the seeds is diluted, and the bird population increases.

able in this condition, especially since vitamin E is said to produce some antiestrogenic effect.

Estrogen can also affect the balance of rennin (an enzyme that plays an important part in the maintenance of blood pressure) and angiotensin (a peptide that is capable of causing constriction of the blood vessels). Rennin causes increased amounts of angiotensin to be produced, which results in high blood pressure.

3. PMS-A (ALLERGY)

Almost the entire spectrum of symptoms may be caused by an underlying, undiagnosed, or masked allergy or intolerance to common foods or chemicals.

Hypersensitivities of this kind are often, but not always, mediated via the immune system, and standard allergy profile tests are a good start in the diagnostic process. However, the standard tests should not be the final diagnosis unless a series of provocation challenge tests follows.

The most common trigger foods and chemicals appear to be yeast, wheat, gluten, milk, and house dust, although I have seen cases of

---

Foods High in Vitamin E

egg	parsley
lettuce	peanuts
margarine	salmon steak
mayonnaise	sweet potato
milk	vegetables (dark-green
oils, cold-pressed	leafy ones)

Food High in Vitamin B$_{15}$ (Pangamic Acid)

almonds	rice bran
apricot kernels	rice shoots
liver	yeast (brewer's)

PMS-A patients who were hypersensitive to their own lipstick or perfume or some common foods such as lettuce and potato.

4. PMS-C (CANDIDA)

Thrush (monilia), a common condition caused by a yeast fungus called *Candida albicans*, is responsible for a great many health problems. I have seen more women who suffer from premenstrual syndrome because of systemic candidiasis than almost any other single group.

These women should be treated for the underlying thrush by avoiding all alcohol and yeast-containing foods and being kept under observation for PMS symptoms. If the PMS symptoms do not disappear, one should begin to look for other possible causes for their menstrual problems.

5. PMS-H (HYPOGLYCEMIA)

These patients tend to suffer from wild fluctuations in blood-sugar levels. They are often very tired and feel dizzy and mentally confused, especially on awakening and in midafternoon. Their symptoms tend to be worse when they do not eat, and they are susceptible to sugar binges.

The most common symptoms and signs of this group are the timing and severity of their attacks in relation to the amount of food, especially sweets, that they eat. They can be prone to fainting spells and often cry for no apparent reason, mimicking classic neurotic symptoms. Of course, hypoglycemia can be determined from a glucose-tolerance test.

Sufferers are particularly sensitive to sugars and often have excessive insulin activity. Garlic, chromium, and yeast supplements affect insulin activity and may aggravate this condition.

PMS-H sufferers are invariably deficient in magnesium and need strong supplements of zinc and vitamin B_3. Zinc aids the synthesis and release of gamma linoleic acid (GLA), which reduces symptoms of PMS in general. Vitamin B_3 is used in the conversion of GLA into prostaglandin (PGE 1), which is a hormone-like substance that helps with the physical and mental symptoms of premenstrual syndrome.

Apart from breast milk, the oil of evening primrose is one of the best sources of linoleic acid and GLA. This is probably one of the reasons why this supplement has proven so helpful in the treatment of premenstrual syndrome.

Some researchers have suggested that ample amounts of unrefined grains and legumes can be helpful; however, our clinical experience has shown that this can sometimes be counterproductive. First of all, many patients have an intolerance to grain, especially bran, wheat, and corn, and second, some of these products, such as the legumes, are particularly high in phytic acid, which blocks the absorption of zinc. Zinc supplements taken on an empty stomach can help to circumvent this problem.

Each case is different because people may be intolerant to some foods and not others. An intolerance tends to irritate the gut walls, and this will also cause problems with absorption.

Allergens and Addictions

The list of potential allergens is endless, but apart from toxic chemicals, the most common offenders are corn, wheat, sugar, coffee, chocolate, milk, malt, barley, and yeast.

If you look at the foods listed above carefully, you will notice that they are probably some of the most common ingredients that we use. We eat them very frequently, often without realizing we are eating them so often. For example, sausage may contain wheat, salt may contain sugar, commercial fruit juices often contain yeast.

It is possible to become addicted to a substance because it is eaten too often or in large quantities. Most if not all of the common food allergies are masked because they are actually addictions.

As soon as the withdrawal symptoms start, one eats the offending food again and thereby successfully masks the allergy. Coffee addicts, chocaholics, and cigarette smokers all feel better after ingesting their toxin. So beware, because often the allergic food is one you actually like and eat a lot of.

Hypoglycemics tend to fare better on a high-protein diet, but they should avoid excessive fats. Animal meats contain antibiotics and estrogen, and both these factors can aggravate hypoglycemic sufferers.

One way to get around some of these problems is to include spirulina in a dietary regimen that consists of small snacks with a good balance of vegetables and nonallergenic grains, such as brown rice and millet. Spirulina contains all the necessary amino acids without being derived from animal sources.

6. PMS-D (DEPRESSION)

This group is characterized by severe premenstrual depression and, at times, suicidal tendencies. In most cases one of the first practical things to do is to administer a Hoffer and Osmond diagnostic test to ascertain the possibility of suicide and to quantitatively define the role of estrogen in the depression. The test also helps to discover if the patient has an underlying psychiatric problem that is mistaken for, and often masked by, premenstrual syndrome.

Some of these patients may benefit from oral contraceptives because they tend to have a relatively high progesterone/estrogen ratio. They are invariably deficient in or dependent on B-complex vitamins, especially vitamin B_6, and magnesium.

Heavy-metal intoxication, especially by lead, is common, and many of these women find they are worse after physical exercise—especially jogging in a city. This is partly because they pass more polluted air through their lungs and partly because the decreased postexertion pH of body fluids tends to leach lead into the bloodstream.

Copper is also a factor because it may indirectly cause a lowering of some neurotransmitters in the brain.

PMS-D sufferers are probably the only premenstrual syndrome patients for whom we sometimes recommend tryptophan, and when this is done we often add DL-phenylalanine and tyrosine to the supplement regimen.

They are usually negatively affected by any forms of stress (the "I can't cope" syndrome), but their adrenal involvement varies greatly. Many suffer from hypoadrenocorticism (adrenal exhaustion) and benefit from additional supplements of vitamin B and Siberian gin-

Foods High in Zinc

beef	mushrooms
bran	oatmeal
Brazil nuts	oysters
crab	pork
egg	pumpkin seeds
grains	rice, brown
herring	sunflower seeds
kidney	tuna
lamb	veal
milk	yeast (brewer's)

Foods High in Magnesium

almonds	lima beans
apricots, dried	molasses
avocado	oatmeal
baked beans	peaches
barley	peanuts
beef	peas
Brazil nuts	pecans
carrots (raw)	pork
cashews	potato
chicken	rice
citrus fruits	sesame
corn	soybeans
crab	tomato (raw)
dates	vegetables (dark-
fish (flounder,	green leafy ones)
salmon, tuna)	wheat germ
lentils	

seng. A careful history check and some specialized tests can often single out this group.

Some, however, suffer from excessive adrenal stimulation, especially during the early phases of the syndrome, which in any case often precedes adrenal exhaustion. Vitamin B_5, ginseng, and excessive vitamin C may actually produce a temporary worsening of the symptoms when the adrenal glands are overstimulated. One of the clues is that these patients are very cyclic in their responses to stress, which can vary from the need for total isolation and avoidance of sensory inputs (they do not even like to talk at the time) to the need for mental or physical stimulation.

7. PMS-F (FLUID RETENTION)

Although this group shares many signs and symptoms with sufferers of PMS-E, the underlying hormonal-metabolic mechanism may be quite different.

Fluid retention, abdominal and breast swelling, weight gain, and cravings for salty and/or sweet foods are common to both groups. However, menstrual blood is less often clotty, and tiredness is not a predominant feature.

Often excessive alcohol intake and decreased liver function exist along with a degree of hyperinsulinism in these patients. They are often under continuous, although not necessarily excessive stress, which triggers the increased secretion of aldosterone. Because aldosterone is a stress hormone that causes the body to retain sodium, more fluid will be retained.

We know that some PMS-F sufferers are deficient in dopamine which in turn may affect sodium and magnesium balance. For this reason tyrosine and DL-phenylalanine may prove useful.

Dietary Guidelines

Almost all cases of premenstrual syndrome respond favorably to oil of evening primrose, magnesium, zinc, vitamin E, and vitamin B_6 supplementation. In some cases, the vitamin ratios have to be altered. Fluid retention, for instance, does not appear to be influenced by oil of evening primrose, while it seems to respond well to vitamin B_6.

Following are some basic dietary guidelines:

- People who produce excessive estrogen and suffer from subclinical hypothyroidism may benefit from avoiding members of the cabbage family (Brussels sprouts, cauliflower, soybeans, peanuts) and animal meats, especially red meat.

- All sufferers of premenstrual syndrome should restrict high-sugar foods, including honey, dried fruit, undiluted fruit juices, and sweet desserts.

- Take plenty of vitamin C, vitamin B_6, and magnesium and also a little zinc (5 milligrams per day).

- Take a good vitamin B-complex supplement but avoid those that contain too much folic acid (no more than 50 micrograms) and excessive PABA (no more than 50 milligrams).

- Alcohol, coffee, tea, chocolate, and salt intake should be as low as possible.

- Be very wary of adopting a specific restrictive diet, especially if it varies greatly from your usual one. Before changing your diet, examine the possibility of food intolerances and allergies, because there is no point in being free of premenstrual syndrome if you end up with an irritable colon.

The Good Oil: Oil of Evening Primrose

When English physician Dr. Caroline Shreeve ended up in the divorce court because her extreme irritability had made it impossible for her to get along with her husband, she decided to look at the reasons for her behavior. For the previous five years she had suffered extreme symptoms of premenstrual syndrome.

Dr. Shreeve decided it was time to look for a possible cure. She tried everything: fluid and salt restrictions— "helpful, but not enough"; yoga and relaxation— "wonderful at most times, but during PMS many women don't feel like doing anything that sensible"; vitamin therapy— "certainly an integral part of any successful treatment, but not sufficient for many people"; diuretics— "they can cause more trouble than they are worth"; progesterone—

"very useful, but not all women who should respond to this treatment do so"; the pill— "too many worries about side effects"; tranquilizers— "they achieve nothing"; and vitamin B₆—"useful only in those who are deficient in this vitamin to start with." Dr. Shreeve was getting nowhere fast.

In 1981 Dr. Shreeve married again, this time to a psychotherapist, and during the same year, she attended an international medical symposium where she heard Dr. Michael Brush of the St. Thomas Hospital, London, talk about a series of double-blind, crossover trials in the use of a flower for the treatment of premenstrual syndrome! To be more precise, it was with the extract of a bright yellow English flower called the evening primrose (*Oenothera biennis*). Its seeds are crushed and produce an oil that is a rich source of a rare essential fatty acid called gamma linoleic acid (GLA). (One of the few natural sources of GLA is breast milk.)

Essential fatty acids, or polyunsaturates, contain the active ingredient linoleic acid, from which the body makes GLA. However, as soon as a polyunsaturated oil is heated, deodorized, hydrogenated, or otherwise artificially processed, the linoleic acid is changed into a "bad oil" form, which actually blocks further synthesis of GLA.

In addition, the synthesis of GLA can be blocked by a diet that is high in animal fats and alcohol and low in zinc, magnesium, or vitamin B₆, as well as the presence of viral infections and diabetes.

GLA is converted into prostaglandin (PGE 1), which is a ubiquitous hormone-like substance that helps to reduce blood pressure, prevent inflammations, activate insulin, produce a sense of well-being in many people, and relieve the physical and mental symptoms of premenstrual syndrome.

In fact, Dr. Shreeve claims that a deficiency of GLA is one of the main causes of premenstrual syndrome and other symptoms associated with this syndrome. She also claims that the "good oil" can reduce cholesterol levels, lower blood pressure, improve eczema, fix brittle nails, reduce the severity of hangovers, and help in the treatment of hyperactivity. It has been used experimentally in the treatment of multiple sclerosis.

Dr. Shreeve has since written a book on premenstrual syndrome called *Premenstrual Syndrome, the Curse That Can Be Cured.*

HYPERACTIVITY AND CHILDREN'S LEARNING DIFFICULTIES

CHAPTER 8

One of the difficult factors in understanding hyperactivity is distinguishing true hyperactive behavior from the normal restlessness and curiosity of children.

While it is true that some of the symptoms of hyperactivity can be a normal extension of behavior patterns, it is also clear that some children are being adversely affected by environmental and lifestyle factors. The difficulties experienced by these children and their parents make hyperactivity a distressing and serious problem, but one that can be cured.

Any form of abnormal behavior, such as hyperactivity, can be the result of an enormous range of factors: emotional stress, difficult or restrictive environments, psychological or physical abuse. These and other psychodynamic possibilities should be properly evaluated by a competent professional, usually a child psychiatrist or psychologist. There is, however, a growing body of scientific evidence that shows that exposure to commonly used chemicals (including food additives), some nutrients, and poor nutrition can cause allergies or intolerances in children.

Unfortunately, these allergies and intolerances not only cause behavioral problems but can also influence a child's ability to learn. Thus it is not uncommon to find that hyperactive children tend to be slow learners. Paradoxically, this happens in spite of the fact that such children are usually very intelligent.

Do you find this difficult to believe? Just imagine you were trying to read a legal paper or a scientific article while someone was tickling your ear or feet with a feather. The constant neurological distraction of the tickling would make it very difficult for you to concentrate and comprehend what you were reading, irrespective of how intelligent you are! Allergies or intolerances to food and sensitivities to chemicals act in the same way: they constantly irritate the child's nervous system and make it difficult for him to concentrate and learn.

Hyperactivity and Heredity

Heredity cannot be ruled out as a factor contributing to hyperactivity. The boy-girl ratio for hyperactivity is eight to one, and some psychiatrists think that more boys suffer from food sensitivity because it is passed on to children via the mother's X chromosome, especially if it is a case of defective enzymes.

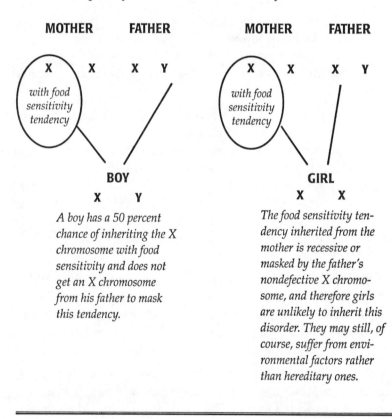

MOTHER   FATHER

X (with food sensitivity tendency)   X   X   Y

BOY
X   Y

A boy has a 50 percent chance of inheriting the X chromosome with food sensitivity and does not get an X chromosome from his father to mask this tendency.

MOTHER   FATHER

X (with food sensitivity tendency)   X   X   Y

GIRL
X   X

The food sensitivity tendency inherited from the mother is recessive or masked by the father's nondefective X chromosome, and therefore girls are unlikely to inherit this disorder. They may still, of course, suffer from environmental factors rather than hereditary ones.

Signs and Symptoms

Many hyperactive children tend to display some degree of anxiety or depression and are often tense. Sometimes these children are lethargic, tend to sleep or lie down doing nothing for hours, even days on end, only to emerge from their lethargy behaving very aggressively and destructively for no apparent reason.

HYPERACTIVITY

Nervous System Symptoms

- Hyperactive, wild, unrestrained, inattentive, disruptive
- Talkative
- Short attention span
- Clumsiness, tremor, uncoordination
- Restless legs, finger tapping
- Insomnia, nightmares, inability to fall asleep
- Nervous, irritable, upset, short-tempered
- High strung, excitable, agitated
- Moody, tired, weak, exhausted, listless
- Depressed
- Easily moved to tears, easily hurt
- Highly sensitive to odor, light, sound, pain, and/or cold

Other Medical Symptoms

- Stuffy or watery nose, sneezing, nose rubbing
- Aches in head, back, neck muscles: "growing pains" or aches not related to exercise
- Stomach problems, nausea, upset stomach, bad breath
- Gassy stomach, belching
- Bloating, vomiting
- Diarrhea, constipation
- Bladder problems, daytime or nighttime bedwetting, urgency, burning or pain with urine
- Pale or dark circles or puffiness below eyes
- Swollen glands or lymph nodes in neck
- Ear problems, repeated fluid behind eardrums, ringing ears
- Dizziness
- Excessive perspiration, low-grade fever

Behavioral Signs and Symptoms

Rocks crib and knocks head during infancy

Is aggressive and/or disruptive at home and school

Touches everything and everybody

Disturbs other children

Does not respond to discipline

Behaves unpredictably

Panics easily

Throws tantrums

Is impatient—wants things now!

Fidgets

Cannot sit still

Does not finish projects

Wears out furniture, toys, etc.

Is destructive

Fights with other children

Refuses to follow directions

Is clumsy—has difficulty fastening buttons or tying shoelaces

Usually very intelligent but has difficulties learning

Hard to put to bed and sleep

Wakes up early

Lies

Wets bed

Sometimes has speech difficulties

Some of the children are quite allergic and suffer from runny noses, throat mucus, sinusitis, hay fever, asthma, skin rashes, and digestive problems such as loose bowels, diarrhea, and constipation. They often display abdominal bloating after eating, and their eyes tend to be watery and sometimes red and sore, especially on awakening.

Not every hyperactive child exhibits all, or even the majority, of these symptoms, but if enough of them are present, your child may suffer from hyperactivity.

Causes

SENSITIVITY TO FOOD ADDITIVES

Probably the best known scientist involved in research on the causes of hyperactivity was Dr. Ben Feingold of the Kaiser Permanente Medical Center in San Francisco, California. In the 1960s Dr. Feingold discovered that some chemicals added to our food could provoke a reaction in susceptible children that manifests itself as hyperactive behavior.

Dr. Feingold claimed he had irrefutably proved a cause-and-effect relationship between food additives and hyperactive behavior. The most convincing proof was the ability to switch off and then provoke the reaction in hyperactive children by withholding and later readministering the offending substance.

Millions of children all over the world have gone on the "Feingold diet" and benefited from it. This diet consists of eliminating all foods that are colored, preserved, canned, instant, or are known to contain chemical additives. At the same time, all foods containing the natural salicylates are also avoided. This is because Dr. Feingold discovered that many children are unusually sensitive to a chemical "cousin" of salicylate (the common ingredient in aspirin), which is found in some fruits and vegetables, including almonds, apples, apricots, blackberries, cloves, cucumbers, pickles, currants, gooseberries, raisins, mint flavors, nectarines, oranges, peaches, plums, prunes, raspberries, strawberries, teas of any kind, tomatoes, and oil of wintergreen.

Red Food Coloring

While working on the problem of irritation caused by flea bites, Dr. Feingold found that colorings, especially red ones, were a major factor in hyperactive behavior. This is not as bizarre as it sounds, because cochineal, the traditional red cake coloring, was made from the crushed bodies of tiny cactus-eating insects. It is the secretions made in the flea's body that cause most of the irritation when one is bitten.

The Feingold diet is responsible for curing up to about 40 percent of hyperactive children and helping as many as 60 percent. However, it is also a fact that many children fail to respond, or respond only partially, to this regimen.

What, then, is the reason for this failure rate? At the time of Dr. Feingold's research, other scientists were busy looking into the role played by nutrients, smells, fumes, heavy metals, and other substances in altering human behavior. Several scientists in the United States, Europe, and Australia were becoming aware of a greater range of possible factors.

HYPOGLYCEMIA

It has been found that a large number of hyperactive children suffer from abnormal fluctuations in their blood-sugar levels; they are hypoglycemic.

Hypoglycemia means "low blood sugar" and results when sugars, refined carbohydrates, or other blood-sugar-elevating substances are eaten (especially on an empty stomach). The body overreacts by producing chemicals that send blood-sugar levels plummeting. For a number of reasons the blood sugar may fail to return to normal levels unless further amounts of sweets are eaten. During this period, while levels are low, the individual is in a state of biochemical stress. Very much like a drug addict or alcoholic, they need another shot. Often these people are classified as "sugarholics"—they are addicted to substances that elevate their blood sugar.

All these metabolic ups and downs unsettle the nervous system and can cause a variety of behavioral symptoms, including hyperactivity. They often make it impossible for the child to concentrate or study, and the child quickly falls behind in school work.

It is important to understand that, in some individuals, blood sugar may drop from a high level to a reasonably normal level so fast that the nervous system is adversely affected. Also, what is a normal level for one individual may be too low for another.

The other essential point is that although sugar may trigger the drop, any substance to which the individual is sensitive (allergic or intolerant) may cause blood-sugar levels to fall. Sometimes people suffering from this problem show symptoms opposite to hyperactivity. They are always tired, sleepy, and lethargic and never get anything done.

SENSITIVITIES TO MOLDS, FUNGI, FERMENTS, AND YEASTS

It was then found that quite a few hyperactive children were also hypersensitive or allergic to fungi. After they were placed on a yeast-free or mold-free diet and given antifungals when needed and their environment was cleared of mold, the children were tested and desensitized. Only then did their behavior improve.

MINERAL DEFICIENCIES OR IMBALANCES

This can be caused by excessive ingestion of or contamination by minerals.

Excessive copper can come from drinking water (via copper piping) or from food (via copper saucepans), leading to a relative deficiency of zinc (because zinc competes with copper for absorption). Copper generally tends to increase nervous excitation, whereas zinc has a calming effect. Frozen vegetables are usually deficient in zinc, and vegetarian diets that have too many soya beans can boost copper to unacceptable levels.

Double-blind Tests

By 1950, Dr. William Crook, another leading figure in environmental allergies, was performing the first of the double-blind studies in this area with a young patient who had a problem with milk.

In a double-blind test, nobody—patient, parents, or doctor—knows which medication is the placebo and which is the suspect substance.

In this case, Dr. Crook's patient felt quite well for the first two weeks (while taking the placebo), but after changing to the second group of tablets (the ones containing milk), symptoms such as stuffy nose, fatigue, stomachaches, headaches, depression, and irritability reappeared within three days.

HEAVY METAL INTOXICATION

There are some people so sensitive to certain fumes and odors that it causes them to behave strangely. I can recall one case where a child was affected by his father's aftershave lotion.

More common sources of irritation can be gas stoves, aerosol sprays, perfumes, and, of course, lead from exhaust fumes. Is your child's playground by a busy main road or, worse still, at an intersection? Do you buy fruit and vegetables from street-corner markets? If so, these may be sources of unwanted heavy metals.

SENSITIVITY TO INHALED CHEMICALS

Deodorant sprays, hairsprays, oven cleaners, and dozens of commonly used household products and substances found in your child's school may be causing an allergic reaction and hyperactive symptoms.

Treatment

Many hyperactive children may be able to eat some or all of the fruits and vegetables excluded by the Feingold diet after they have eliminated some of the other contributing factors discussed under "Causes."

It seems that so many allergies or intolerances happen because of a combination of factors. If a child is allergic to mold, dust, or pollens, the sensitivity to salicylates may be reduced dramatically after these other allergies have been taken care of. The opposite is also true. A child who continues to eat something to which he or she is allergic is more likely to exhibit symptoms when exposed to pollens or other airborne factors.

Once placed on the appropriate diet, many of those allergic children can tolerate some exposure to dust, pollens, and other substances without being severely affected. In many cases, when a sensitivity has been established, it is possible that the child will lose it after several months. This is more common with foods or inhalant allergies than with chemical food additives.

It is sometimes possible to desensitize sufferers with allergy drops under the tongue, whereas at other times a neutralization technique known as serial titration is called for.

Serial titration is carried out by provoking the symptoms with an extract of the suspect substance and then progressively diluting the extract. Each dilution is given to the patient to ascertain if it can switch off or neutralize the symptoms. If it fails to do so, it is further diluted until a dilution of the extract is found that is capable of stopping the symptom. A vaccine is then prepared and is taken by the patient to neutralize the allergy.

After a suitable time, some of these children are able to start eating the offending foods on a four-day rotation diet—the food can be eaten once every four days.

I want to make it very clear that all I have said so far must not be taken to mean that hyperactivity is a case of "either-or." While it is not uncommon for a hyperactive child to be either hypoglycemic, sensitive to chemicals, sensitive to gluten, or allergic to environmental factors, each of these can be just one factor in the whole problem. It can often happen that an individual has several sensitivities or

Junk Food and Hypoglycemia

In a series of tests at a school for problem children in the western suburbs of Sydney—an area renowned for high levels of air pollution and children with allergies, asthma, and learning difficulties—more than 75 percent of children tested were found to be hypoglycemic.

When these fluctuations were leveled out by eliminating junk foods and sugars from the diet and supplementing vitamin C, vitamin B, magnesium, and zinc, most of the children improved remarkably. Another series of investigations found these children to be equally sensitive to fructose (the sugar commonly found in fruits) and to sucrose (cane sugar). A small number were found to react badly to dried fruits.

A diet eliminating all sugars, including honey and dried fruits, helped a considerable number of hyperactive children. Meanwhile, quite coincidentally, another suspect substance was uncovered—yeast.

allergies. In some cases, every one of the suspect substances has to be eliminated before the child will function normally again. In other cases, taking care of the major ones will sufficiently enhance the body's own ability to overcome the remaining sensitivities to a point where they do not cause any symptoms.

Above all, a thorough evaluation is mandatory for each case. Remember, every one of us is a unique individual, biochemically as well as psychologically.

THE FEINGOLD DIET

After you have removed all foods with artificial colorings and flavorings from your child's diet, as Dr. Feingold recommends on page 123, the next step is to check on common everyday foods, as these may be involved in a masked intolerance.

Skin allergy tests are not very helpful in identifying food sensitivities, although they are useful in detecting allergies to pollen, house dust, mites, animal dandruff, and other inhaled substances. Intradermal and sublingual tests are much more likely to indicate food sensitivities, with the added advantage that the therapist is then able to prepare desensitizing vaccines (drops) or another neutralizing therapy.

Milk, as most parents have heard, is a very popular suspect allergen, and it is closely followed by grains, especially gluten-containing ones

---

Masked Intolerances: What Are They?

An intolerance or allergy can be masked by continual intake of the allergenic substance. If you are addicted to anything, every time you take another dose you will feel better because you avoid the withdrawal symptoms.

The addiction masks the reality that the substance is toxic to you. In the same way, eating something you are allergic to several times each day will tend to mask the symptoms of the allergic reaction. This does not apply to everyone who is allergic, but if it does, the individual will not be aware that he or she is allergic.

like wheat, rye, oats, and malt. Other foods such as sugar, peas, beans, citrus fruits, beef, pork, chicken, and potato may also be problems. By eliminating these foods one at a time, you may find that your child's symptoms improve by the fourth or fifth day, but if not, persevere for up to three weeks.

To find out exactly which foods have been causing problems, introduce them one at a time to see whether the symptoms return. There are tests that can be done by trained practitioners, but they are fairly controversial in the eyes of orthodox physicians. They include the now very old and unreliable cytotoxic test, the RAST test, the pulse test, and the kinesiology test.

OLIGOANTIGENIC DIET

A simple way to determine whether your child is suffering from a food allergy is to adopt a strict elimination diet called an oligoantigenic diet.

Place the child on basic multivitamin and mineral supplements plus a little zinc and magnesium. Then continue with a strict diet that excludes potentially allergenic foods. The basis of the diet includes food such as sweet potatoes, cabbage, carrots, free-range lamb or turkey, pears, and purified water. After a few weeks you should be able to notice the change in the child's behavior.

Once you have established that the child is better, start to reintroduce foods—one per day. Leave wheat and grain products, yeast, and sugar until last. If any food is responsible or even a contributing factor, you will know by the change in the child's behavior. This is one way you can establish which are safe foods and which are not.

Preventative Measures

One way to lessen the possibility of your child acquiring a food allergy or intolerance is to practice preventative medicine and take precautions during pregnancy.

The following steps will help you to establish the best possible environment for your child during pregnancy and childhood.

DURING PREGNANCY

It is very important to eat a well-balanced diet. Vary your diet and avoid eating large quantities of any single food, especially those you dislike or those that disagree with you. A varied diet also helps build up digestive enzymes for passing on to your baby through breast milk.

There is some evidence from Sweden that if you are sensitive to milk, it will probably upset your baby as well. Calcium is needed during pregnancy, and if you cannot drink milk, it is available in yogurt, some vegetables, and certain hard cheeses.

If you find that you are craving a certain type of food, it is usually an indication that your diet is deficient in a vitamin or mineral found in that food. It is necessary to take a good look at what you are eating, and it may be advisable to consider taking vitamin and mineral supplements. Also remember that vegetables will lose fewer vitamins and minerals when they are juiced than when they are cooked.

AFTER YOUR CHILD IS BORN

It is very important to breastfeed. Try to arrange for your baby to be put onto your breast as soon as possible after the birth so that she or he benefits from the colostrum, the thickish yellow substance that comes from the nipples just before milk starts flowing. Colostrum plays a very important part in helping to build up protective bacteria in the baby's digestive tract, and it also gives some immune protection.

Do not begin feeding your baby solids too soon. Cereal is liable to be a major hazard, since it generally contains wheat, and most canned baby dinners contain wheat flour as a thickener. There has, however, been a healthy move toward reducing sugar, salt, and monosodium glutamate in most baby food products. If you suspect your baby may be prone to food allergies or sensitivities, avoid chocolate and egg until the baby is nine months or older.

If weaning to cow's milk or cow's milk formula causes diarrhea or any other adverse symptoms, remove it from the baby's diet completely until the symptoms subside. This also goes for yogurt, puddings, and probably even cheese. If your baby has difficulty with cow's milk and you are not breastfeeding, vegetable juices such as carrot juice, nut and seed milks, and goat's milk are good alternative sources of calcium.

It is very important to give your baby a wide variety of natural foods and to avoid processed or canned foods. Rotate and diversify your baby's diet as much as possible because a food allergy or intolerance is much more likely to develop if a food is taken every day.

It is true that babies are initially wary of new foods. However, you cannot mistake real, determined dislike. No matter how wholesome a food is, do not persevere with it if it is causing distress. This is how hidden or masked allergies start.

NEUROTOXINS: POLLUTION, CHEMICALS, AND YOUR BRAIN

CHAPTER 9

The diagnosis of human illness is, in many ways, an exercise in the detection of biochemical, psychological, or physiological disturbances in an individual. People only become aware of the effects of such disturbances when symptoms of this disturbance become apparent. Symptoms are the body's own warning signals that tell us something is amiss.

We become ill for many different reasons: stress, trauma, malignant cells, infectious agents (viruses, bacteria, fungi, etc.), or simply because we do not receive sufficient nutrients to enable our body to ward off an attack. Whatever the causes, symptoms can vary greatly from person to person and from illness to illness. Of course, the symptoms one actually feels can have their origin in different parts of the body.

We tend to think of body functions only in terms of the organs responsible for them. Because of the particular orientation of orthodox medical education, physicians often think of organ functions as if each were a separate entity. We talk about heart functions, kidney functions, and lung functions, almost as if these organs existed as independent, self-contained units. But, in fact, each organ is totally dependent on every other organ. For example, it is pointless to talk about heart disease as if the heart existed in total isolation. The heart's blood supply depends on healthy circulation, and blood is useless unless it is full of the necessary ingredients for life—nutrients from the foods we eat, the gases we breathe, and the fluids we drink. To some extent, our circulation is also dependent on physical activity, which can be affected by anything from our sex life to our working conditions.

Brain functions are largely regulated by the hormones the brain produces from amino acids present in the food we eat, and the brain cannot get these unless the foods are digested and absorbed. However, the brain is a very delicate organ, and its intricate hormonal system can become unbalanced; its synchronicity can be thrown out of kilter; and its regulatory neurotransmitter chemicals can be antagonized, deactivated, or inhibited by a considerable number of substances—natural or otherwise.

There is a particular class of chemicals called neurotoxins that can damage the nervous system and can, therefore, cause almost any emotional or behavioral symptom—from hallucinations to depression, from sleeplessness to dementia, and from memory loss to psychosis.

Changes brought about by neurotoxins are so subtle and treacherous that most people who are affected by them have no idea what is causing their symptoms. Often their doctors are equally unaware of the real cause of the problem, and they begin to search for physical causes for each of the symptoms that might, in fact, be the early warnings of neurotoxicity.

Tingling and numbness of the fingers or toes, slight tremors or a shaky feeling, slight uncoordination, impotence, and decreased sensations of touch are all characteristics of neurotoxicity. Later, perhaps years after the initial exposure to a neurotoxin, there may be some general pains, problems with vision, a decreased sense of smell and taste, lowered alertness, loss of memory, lethargy, irritability, and even depression, hallucinations, or psychosis—or a combination of any of these.

In some cases, a few of these effects are irreversible because of the difficulties of repairing or replacing damaged or lost cells. The consequences on the human brain are therefore almost invariably permanent. Because the nature of the presenting symptoms are so diverse, these are often attributed to an excessive workload, advancing age, or even stress. Let us now take a look at some of the neurotoxins in our environment.

Ethoxyethanol

This is a widely used industrial solvent related to the alcohol found in lacquers, dyes, varnish removers, and many other industrial processes. It has always been regarded as safe, and indeed, when the compound was extensively tested in laboratory animals, it was shown to produce no toxic effects. Even pregnant rats did not suffer when exposed to doses equivalent to half the allowable limits. But their offspring did! Subsequent tests showed significant changes in brain chemistry and after-birth behavior.

The implications of the following experiment are also quite interesting. B. K. Nelson, a scientist at the National Institute for Occupational Safety and Health in America, gave a group of pregnant rats the same amount of ethoxyethanol, which had been shown to be safe for them but toxic to their offspring. At the same time he mixed a little alcohol

Pollution and Learning Difficulties in Children

Children are particularly susceptible to toxins of all kinds. Because learning is such an essential part of growing up, the effects of pollution on brain functions can be devastating in a child.

Usually the first signs are what we would normally call altered behavior, but behavior is such an individualistic phenomenon that few parents (or even teachers) are aware of the problem until it is too late.

The Select Committee on Nutrition and Human Needs of the United States Senate 95th Congress on June 22, 1977 stated:

> The early symptoms of lead poisoning are subtle, subjective, and non-specific, and therefore not so easily recognized in children. In children such mild symptoms are often either overlooked or attributed to other diseased states, so that poisoning due to lead is more likely to be recognized first at a late, or severe stage on the basis of nervous system involvement.

In other words, by the time we are aware that our children are suffering from subtle pollutants it may be too late.

into their drinking water. He discovered that the effects of this combination on the brain neurochemistry of their offspring were twice as severe as those caused by ethoxyethanol alone.

There are rather frightening implications because of this phenomenon. It is quite possible that a great many people who are infrequently exposed to small amounts of ethoxyethanol may suffer no symptoms—at least no observable ones—from such exposure. However, if the same people consume regular amounts of alcohol in addition to being exposed to ethoxyethanol, although they are not directly harmed, the toxicity of ethoxyethanol is such that their children may suffer serious neurological consequences.

Carbon Disulfide

Discovered in the latter part of the 18th century, carbon disulfate (CS_2) was originally used as a general anesthetic. In 1840 J. Simpson, a Scottish surgeon, reported that he was no longer using CS_2 because it caused hallucinations, headaches, and nausea in his patients. Within a few years CS_2 was used extensively as a solvent in industrial processes. It was then discovered that CS_2 could "soften" rubber at any temperature, thus making it possible to manufacture many things such as raincoats, rubber toys, and balloons. Of course, anyone working with this substance was exposed to its deadly fumes.

Already by 1856 the writings of the Frenchman Dr. Auguste Delpeech contained a warning:

> He who works in the "sulphur" is no longer a man. He may still make a living from day to day in unskilled labor. He will never be able to establish an independent position for himself. The depressing influence of the carbon sulphide upon his willpower, the painful consequences of his indifference, and the loss of his memory, prevent him from entering another occupation.

The doctor also described how some of the workers' children, who spent a few days playing near their fathers while they worked, were "stricken with a type of raging delirium."

Alan Anderson, writing in *Psychology Today*, tells us that in 1902 a British publication, *Dangerous Trades*, described a factory in which the windows were barred to prevent crazed workers from leaping forth during their frequent delirious attacks! Meanwhile the rubber industry has developed, causing untold thousands of unsuspecting workers to lose their health and sanity.

In Finland, workers in modern, well-ventilated, clean rayon factories have been tested and shown to have lost some neuromuscular speed, intelligence, and psychomotor ability.

Nitrates

Although nitrates themselves are not particularly toxic, when they change to nitrites or nitrosamines they can become quite dangerous. They are suspected of being carcinogenic. Nitrites are capable of causing a condition known as methemoglobinemia—a condition in which blood no longer carries an adequate amount of oxygen. A small child affected with this disease may turn blue and suffer permanent brain damage as a result. As the child grows up, the impairment may show in several ways. Nitrates thus become neurotoxic.

Baby formulas made with well water may have a high content of nitrates. Well water can easily become contaminated by pesticides and other chemicals that are used in agriculture. Sometimes local water supplies can be affected by animal wastes, which can be high in nitrate content. Methemoglobinemia can also be caused by air that has been polluted by vanadium.

Volatile Fuels

According to some studies, workers exposed to jet fuels have poor scores in behavioral tests that demand a high degree of concentration. Statistically, such workers were found to have more psychiatric illnesses and symptoms of depression and neurotic behavior.

Similar results were obtained in studies of people exposed to paint solvents. A Scandinavian study reported in *Psychology Today* (July 1982) revealed that when 52 house painters were studied, they scored lower than controls on tests of intellectual capacity, psychomotor coordination, memory, and reaction time. Totally oblivious of the danger, the workers sometimes washed their hands in methyl-n-butyl ketone, a powerful neurotoxin capable of severely damaging the central nervous system.

Surgeons and other operating theater personnel are often exposed to anesthetic gases that can escape from pressure-relief valves used during operations. Nitrous oxide and halothane, two anesthetic gases, when inhaled in concentrations as low as 50 parts per million and one part per million respectively, can affect short-term memory, visual perception, acuity, and cognitive motor responses—the very skills needed in an operating room!

Mercury

Mercury, or quicksilver, has always been regarded as somewhat magical because of its unique property—it is the only metal to be liquid at room temperature.

Its toxic properties have been well known since medieval times, and it has been used extensively as a poison. It has been said that Napoleon, Ivan the Terrible, and Charles II of England all died of mercury poisoning. Records exist to show that in the year 1700 a citizen of Finale, a small town in Italy, sought an injunction against a factory making mercury chloride because its fumes were killing the inhabitants.

A diagnosis of mercury poisoning is difficult to make. One of the problems is that damage may happen before the symptoms manifest themselves; however, symptoms are not apparent until neurological damage has already occurred. So, unfortunately, the accepted daily intake or exposure is that which is enough to cause symptoms.

An article in Science (177 [1982]: 621) reported that, because fetal tissue is particularly susceptible to damage by chemicals and heavy metals, large doses of mercury were given to pregnant mice to test toxicity. All litters tested were born apparently healthy. They developed well, and there appeared to be no difference between the mercury-injected mice and the untreated ones.

Indeed, when the respective brain sizes and neurotransmitter enzyme content were measured two months after birth, everything appeared quite normal. However, when these animals underwent subsequent behavioral tests, the researchers were in for a rude shock. Mice that had been given the mercury showed aberrant behavior patterns.

Instead of exploring a new piece of territory as the control animals did, the mercury-injected mice sat around listlessly and showed no interest whatsoever in their surroundings. When some of them eventually moved around, they often walked backward! The affected animals also showed a greatly reduced desire to groom themselves. The researchers then put the mice through normal swimming tests. Untreated mice learned to swim, while the mercury-exposed mice swam poorly and periodically lapsed into bouts of neuromuscular incoordination.

Strangely enough, mercury was probably the first metal compound to be employed therapeutically. Hippocrates is believed to have pre-

Heavy Metals and Their Effects

Arsenic: giddiness, headaches, general weakness, fatigue

Boron: restlessness, uncoordination, aggressiveness, jitteriness, disorientation

Cadmium: fatigue, smell dysfunctions and lack of taste, increased heart disease risk

Copper: irritability, poor concentration, hyperactivity

Manganese: psychiatric symptoms (French miners exposed to manganese showed symptoms indistinguishable from schizophrenia)

Mercury: tremors, uncoordination, speech problems, psychiatric problems

Nickel: headaches, insomnia, delirium, irritability

Selenium: dizziness, lassitude, depression, fatigue

Tin: limb weakness, vertigo, photophobia

Pesticides in general: neurological, metabolic, and psychiatric general disturbances

Chlorine: skin rashes, lethargy, allergic reactions

Nitrates: possibly carcinogenic

scribed mercury sulfide as a medication. During the 16th century it was extensively used to treat syphilis, and someone with a sense of humor noted that "a night with Venus might lead to a lifetime with mercury."

Known as a toxic time bomb, dental fillings (which can be made from mercury) can slowly but insidiously poison an individual to the point where his or her immune system is working well below normal. The effects can be wide ranging and lead to all sorts of diseases.

MERCURY AND VEGETARIAN DIET

The people who are most at risk from the effect of mercury poisoning are strict vegetarians or vegans because mercury combines with sulfur-containing proteins.

The principal sources of methionine, one of the main sulfur amino acids, are eggs, meats, fish, poultry, and dairy foods. Diets high in methionine and other sulfur amino acids, which are often made from methionine, afford some protection against mercury poisoning. However, this type of diet places a great strain on the body's reserves of vitamin B_6 (pyridoxine) and this should always be taken as a supplement.

Mercury also affects the body's levels of vitamin C by reducing its level within the brain. One of the therapeutic uses of vitamin C in treating heavy metal intoxication is the ability for this vitamin to form complexes with metals, which are then taken out of the body via the urinary system.

Selenium

Selenium combines with mercury, so a diet or intake of water containing adequate selenium gives some protection.

Selenium itself can be highly poisonous, so dietary supplements are not recommended in large doses unless under supervision. Selenium is, nevertheless, a very important and essential mineral. People who drink water with low selenium content or who otherwise acquire selenium deficiency have been found to be prone to cardiovascular disease. Several reports have also linked cancer with a selenium-

Foods High in Vitamin B₆ (Pyridoxine)

avocado	meat (beef, ham, pork)
barley	milk
beans	molasses
Brazil nuts	oranges
carrot	peanuts
cheese	peas
cow's milk	potato
crab	prunes
egg	rice
fish (cod, halibut, herring,	soybeans
mackerel, salmon,	sunflower seeds
sardines, tuna)	wheat bran
lentils	wheat germ
lima beans	whole-meal flour
liver (pork)	yeast (brewer's)

Foods High in Vitamin C (Ascorbic Acid)

alfalfa	guava
banana	kidney
berries (blueberries,	liver (beef)
gooseberries, rasp-	oysters
berries, strawberries)	peppers (red, green)
Brazil nuts	potato
broccoli	spinach
Brussels sprouts	sweet potato
cabbage	tomatoes
cantaloupe	vegetables (green
citrus fruit	leafy ones)
(lemons, oranges)	watermelon

deficient diet, but an excess intake is just as bad as, and in this case far worse than, taking too little.

We know that selenium can pollute water in areas where selenium-rich soil is irrigated. When animals eat the plants that grow there, the metal damages the fetus and, as with thalidomide, can cause the birth of deformed offspring.

Is Selenium an Essential Mineral or a Toxic Metal?

An editorial article by David Rutolo that appeared in the *International Clinical Nutrition Review* in July 1983 asked, "Is selenium an essential mineral or a toxic metal?" The article reported on a heart condition called "Keshan disease" that caused a large number of deaths in China during the 1970s. Researchers discovered that a major contributing factor to this rare condition was a lack of selenium in the diet, and after a vigorous program of corrective supplements, the disease was practically wiped out.

This, however, is only one half of the story. There was also another incident some 20 years before when a group of inhabitants from five Chinese villages were affected by an endemic disease of unknown origin. This disease caused loss of hair and nails and neurological impairments. When the inhabitants of these villages were moved to another area, the physical symptoms disappeared. Those with neurological symptoms needed a longer time to recover.

At first a corn fungus was suspected; however, selenium toxicity was later demonstrated to be the cause of the disease. Apparently, the outbreak of toxicity followed a drought that caused the failure of a rice crop, thereby forcing the villagers to eat more vegetables and maize, which were high in selenium, and fewer protein foods (*American Journal of Clinical Nutrition*).

Selenium levels in the hair, blood, and urine reflect the selenium status of the population. The villagers with selenium toxicity had hair selenium levels 100 times higher than usual and 400 times higher than the people in the selenium-deficient areas where the Keshan disease occurred.

Sulfur supplements do not necessarily provide a shield against the mercury-induced catastrophe because an effective antidote must provide the body with a sulfur-containing protein, not inorganic sulfur.

Pesticides

Pesticides encompass a great number of agents including insecticides, fungicides, fumigants, and rodenticides.

The first pesticide to be commonly used was not the invention of some perverse chemist but one of the ancient Chinese. Called pyrethrum, it was brought to Europe from China by Marco Polo in the 13th century. Although pyrethrum is a natural compound, it is a powerful allergen, and a large number of people are unable to tolerate it. Asthmatics and those suffering from sinusitis seem to be the most easily affected, although I have seen many hyperactive children who appear to be hypersensitive to it.

Probably the most famous pesticide of all is DDT—a chlorinated hydrocarbon that is toxic to the nervous system and does not decompose easily. It can be stored in living tissues for a very long time, and in Australia and other parts of the world, investigators have found that breastfeeding mothers sometimes transmit enormous amounts of pesticides to their infants.

One report, filed by Gregory Miller in 1989, a Griffith University environmental chemist, says that in Queensland breast milk contains 40 times more pesticides than the maximum levels allowed for cow's milk by the World Health Organization.

DDT interferes with calcium absorption, which can result in thin skulls, weak bones, muscular spasms, and mental retardation. DDT is not used much any more, but its replacements are even more dangerous. Most pesticides are now organophosphates, and there are over 150 of them. Organophosphates are a type of insecticide or pesticide specifically toxic to the nerves because they affect acetylcholine, which is the main agent for nerve transmission to muscles. A study set up by the World Health Organization has shown that a diet deficient in acetylcholine will increase a person's susceptibility to the dangers of pesticides. One pesticide in particular, Captan, is almost harmless to a well-nourished person but becomes deadly to someone with a protein-deficient diet.

The type of protein in the diet is also important. Animals raised on soy proteins tend to be deficient in methionine and have a high copper-to-zinc ratio. Such animals are not well protected against mercury poisoning because most antichemical activities in the body need sulfur-containing proteins. If the soybeans have been sprayed with any pesticides, as is often the case, the situation can be quite dangerous.

Soy is also marginally deficient in chromium, another factor that may contribute to ill health if your diet relies heavily on that food. A chromium deficiency affects the body's capacity to make insulin, and this can destabilize the blood-sugar-regulating mechanisms of the body. Rats raised on soy proteins tend to grow poorly and lose their liver reserves of vitamin A when exposed to pesticides.

The Fiber Factor

Although the consumption of high-fiber foods is generally recommended and is normally beneficial to health, it must also be remembered that excessive fiber can cause some proteins to be malabsorbed. If this happens while a person is on a low-protein diet, exposure to pesticides can be fatal. This is an important factor that should be borne in mind when a vegetarian buys a farm for his own use.

Another point worth remembering, especially by those naturopaths who practice extensive fasting therapy, is that most pesticides, especially chlorinated hydrocarbons, accumulate in body fats. During prolonged fasting, these fat stores are broken down for energy, and pesticides, especially DDT, can infiltrate the blood, producing concentrations high enough to become dangerous.

Manganese

Manganese is another potentially toxic metal. It is added to jet fuel to make the outpouring smoke less black—reducing the size of airborne particles so that they tend to disperse without being quite so visible. The particles, however, can penetrate lung tissue and cause serious respiratory and neurological damage.

Manganese is also used in ordinary gasoline as a replacement for lead, but it is doubtful if this is of any health advantage. For example, people employed in the manufacture of dry cell batteries are said to be at risk of developing paralysis as a result of exposure to manganese.

A brochure distributed by a leading hair analysis center in the United States described the symptoms of manganese toxicity as very similar to, if not indistinguishable from, those of schizophrenia, but adds that "symptomatic deficiency of manganese has not been demonstrated in humans."

Paradoxically, the use of manganese is invaluable in counteracting some of the side effects of phenothiazines, a group of psychiatric drugs that produce a syndrome called tardive dyskinesia. When used together with other vitamins, notably niacin, manganese is said to treat this disease quite successfully.

All in all, manganese seems to be a potentially toxic substance that can, nevertheless, be used effectively in the treatment of several diseases. It has been used extensively in orthomolecular psychiatry, but, as I have pointed out, its widespread use as a supplement in high doses is potentially dangerous.

Trichloroethane

This rather frightening-sounding chemical may seem remote but is, in fact, a common thinner used in products such as Liquid Paper. It is one of the milder chlorinated hydrocarbons that acts as a thinner by keeping particles light and easily spreadable.

Hydrocarbons and fluorocarbons can, if inhaled in large enough quantities, cause symptoms similar to those that follow alcohol intoxication. They also cause headaches, ringing in the ears, and hallucinations—not unlike those triggered by LSD. If enough hydrocarbons are inhaled, convulsions and eventually a state of coma may be the unhappy results.

Many people are unwittingly exposed to hydrocarbon and fluorocarbon fumes. Sensitive individuals, especially children, can suffer from twitching muscles and hyperactive reflexes as a result. Those who are hypersensitive or allergic to these compounds may also suffer extreme behavioral disorders because of exposure.

Lighter fluid, correction fluids, fly sprays, paint strippers, and even cough medicines and carsickness pills contain hydrocarbons and fluorocarbons. They can be, and often are, abused by young people seeking a "high."

Toxins and the Environment

Traditional definitions of toxicology for the most part encompass damage to the various body tissues and the likelihood of death. However, in the past few years we have seen the focus shifting to environmental issues and concern with the consequences of long-term exposure to low levels of chemicals. Many scientific investigators, including myself, feel that one of the main criteria in investigating toxicity is that of "functions."

Since function defines life, and since many toxic substances disrupt functions, the effects of exposure should be studied by examining changes in various functions brought about by exposure. Behavioral toxicology is in fact a measurement of subtle functional disorders.

Within this frame of reference, lead poisoning can be seen as a major hazard to behavioral and mental health. A report on lead by the American National Research Council describes the medical and biological effects of environmental pollutants (Select Committee on Nutrition and Human Needs, June 1977) in the following statement:

> The early symptoms of lead poisoning are subtle, subjective, and non-specific, and therefore not so easily recognized in children. In children such mild symptoms are often either overlooked or attributed to other diseased states, so that poisoning due to lead is more likely to be recognized first at a late, or severe stage on the basis of nervous system involvement.

Another example is that of Brethism, which is a syndrome of mercury intoxication characterized by a cluster of symptoms that mimic the behavior of a tormented neurotic:

> I had a sore mouth, dizzy spells, and was so weak and tired at night that I found it hard to get my supper and do my work. I was so grouchy and nervous I would cry at

nothing. . . . I often woke suddenly and had a fluttering feeling like I was scared and floating in space. I was trembly and nervous, and my eyes were bloodshot. I forgot things easily.

A Quick Antipollution Guide

Many of the effects of pollution can be eliminated, avoided, or at least counteracted by sensible approaches and proper nutrition. Following are some alternatives to pollutants used in the home and some ways to help reduce the effect pollutants have on your body.

- Everybody (especially pregnant women and breastfeeding mothers) should try to avoid using pesticides in the home. Pests can be eliminated, or at least minimized, by the judicious use of herbs. Cat thyme, for example, acts as a broad-spectrum insect repellent. The crushed leaves of pennyroyal will help to keep mosquitoes away, and tansy tends to repel flies.

- Vitamin C supplement helps neutralize the effects of nitrates in foods by blocking the formation of potentially dangerous and carcinogenic nitrosamines. The slow release of vitamin C affords some degree of protection from meal to meal and from snacks taken during the day.

- Ozone and nitrogen dioxide, common pollutants in western cities, increase the degeneration of lipid components of lung cells and the subsequent formation of free radicals (these are toxic particles formed during certain chemical reactions in the body and are thought to be responsible for aging, cancer, and degenerative diseases).

- Vitamin C and zinc both inhibit the absorption of lead and help the body dispose of it. Vitamin C also promotes all cellular responses to hormones.

- A lack of calcium or vitamin D_3 predisposes individuals (especially children) to bronchial constriction, which causes breathing difficulties such as asthma.

- The more natural your diet, the less stress you place on your body, and all bodily functions will benefit.

This statement is not from a neurotic person but from a woman who was constantly exposed to mercury in an electric motor components factory. Such symptoms remind us that human behavior reflects the condition of the whole human organism, not just the liver, heart, brain, or an enzyme system. As the study of neurotoxins makes clear, it is the whole organism that complains of pains, becomes confused, or gets irritable and depressed. Hopefully further medical research will be addressed to the study of synergism (combined action) and the less obvious causes of disease.

BEHAVIORAL TOXICOLOGY: POLLUTANTS IN OUR ENVIRONMENT

CHAPTER 10

The theory of evolution may not be accepted by everybody, but it seems evident that the human body has evolved over millions of years and has had to adapt itself to the environment during that time. Originally, although life may have been extraordinarily harsh, the environment was nevertheless quite clean: clean air, a natural diet, plenty of physical activity, and a total absence of manufactured, synthetic substances characterized our ecosystem. The changes that have occurred over very long time spans have allowed for a painstakingly slow, but essential, process of adaptation.

Changes in the Environment

In the past few years we have begun to modify our environment at a frightening and ever-accelerating rate. Dr. Bernard Rimland, a world authority on behavioral toxicology, made the following comments in an address on pollution in San Diego, California: "I use the word 'modify' although on first writing I used the word 'violating,' then considered alternatives such as 'degrading' or 'poisoning' before settling on the ostensibly neutral term 'modify'. I hope my message gets across."

Modern industry is now using more than 100,000 chemicals, of which 575 have already been declared dangerous by the U.S. government. While it is true that many of these chemicals need to be present in reasonably large amounts before they affect our health, there are also some that can cause serious problems at very low levels of exposure.

Most, if not all, chemicals can interact with one another so that their effect becomes greater than the sum of their parts. This is called the "synergistic effect." In practical terms, it simply means that when combined, these can damage our health even at levels considered totally harmless for any of the chemicals alone.

An individual may be capable of coping with two very late nights each and every week without affecting his work output. The same individual may also have the flu once or twice each year, again without suffering any substantial ill effects. But what about if he has the flu and two consecutive late nights? It may just be too much!

Different Types of Pollution

The science that deals with the effects of toxic chemicals on human behavior is named behavioral toxicology, and it is an integral part of orthomolecular medicine and psychiatry.

Among the thousands of cases we see and treat at the Complementary and Environmental Medicine Center, a considerable proportion of so-called psychiatric or behavioral problems, especially among children, are found to be directly or indirectly related to some form of "pollution." I give this word the same meaning as Dr. Rimland:

> Polluted air and water are all too well known. The lesser-known forms, usually not even considered to be manifestations of pollution, are to an increasing degree turning out to be important causes of mental and physical handicap in the human population, especially when the impact occurs during the prenatal or early developmental stages.

> Nutritional pollution includes sins of both omission and commission. It includes the omission from the diet of crucially important vitamins and minerals, especially vitamin C, the B vitamins, as well as vitamin E and such minerals as magnesium, iron, and zinc. The effects are tragic. Foods supplying these nutrients, which are needed for proper health and development, have been replaced with junk foods, gross and damaging amounts of sugar, and other additives that are designed to be attractive to the eye and taste buds, whatever the cost to the rest of the body.

This last statement reminds me of a cartoon I saw once in a magazine that showed a man standing in front of a supermarket shouting, "Come and get it ... beautiful foods ... fresh from the factory!"

Dr. Rimland also tells us that we must include in a list of pollution constituents those factors that could be called inadvertent. These forms of pollution include excess copper from water pipes, lead from auto exhausts, pipes, paints, toothpaste tubes and tinned foods, as well as pesticides and plastics.

Then there is the case of medical pollution. According to Dr. Rimland, medically prescribed and over-the-counter drugs kill more people than breast cancer, while some 50 million hospital-patient days per year are attributable to drug side effects in the United States. And that was in 1975. The numbers have been climbing steadily since, and are currently around 20 percent of all hospital admissions.

Living organisms have a considerable capacity for adaptation, and the human organism has indeed adapted in many ways. For example, as we chew less raw food, our mandibles and teeth have undergone considerable changes, but our capacity to adapt is far from infinite and requires long periods of time.

We all inherit some limitations regarding what foods we can eat. Some of us, for example, lack the suitable enzymes to digest milk, while others acquire limitations for various reasons, ranging from self-imposed restrictions due to religious beliefs to degenerative diseases like diabetes.

Quite apart from these specific limitations, we live in a world that has enough natural poisons without having to cope with the considerable amounts of chemical poisons we have introduced, thus making life even more hazardous than it would naturally be.

Environmental Poisons and Toxicology

Traditionally, toxicology deals with the immediate effects—including death—attributable, directly or indirectly, to ingestion or contact with a poison. However, as a scientific approach, toxicology is not without flaws.

To begin with, most substances are tested singly. The effect of each separate substance is noted, but no allowance is made for the fact that the combined effect of two or three or more chemicals may be quite different from that of a single one. And, when you think of it, this is plain common sense. Mix any two foods or drinks, and you get a taste that is often quite different from that of any of its constituents.

Food additives are tested to see if they produce pathological changes in animals. Blood defects, developmental rates, and certain crucial physiological parameters, such as liver functions, may be examined. From such studies toxicologists calculate quantities of one single substance that can be ingested without causing any measurable abnormality. The resulting figure is then divided by ten to allow for differences among various species, and again by ten for human safety.

This then becomes the allowable daily intake for humans. However, the effects, if any, on the behavior of these animals are almost never measured. Dr. David Ball, director of the National Institute for Environmental Health Sciences, is fond of pointing out that if the effect of thalidomide had been to lower the capacity for academic ability by, say, 10 percent, it would never have been detected.

There is also another very important flaw in the way we test the toxicity of most potential pollutants. Humans are exposed to, and consume, a large amount of chemicals and additives (colorings, preservatives, and so on). The exposed population includes the very young, the very old, the healthy, and the infirm. It also includes the constitutionally strong as well as people with disabilities or predispositions—genetic or otherwise—that may render them more susceptible than others.

Some may have a degree of exposure that is far greater than average. School children are much more likely to eat large amounts of coloring agents from lollipops, popsicles, soft drinks, and similar foods than are adults. Because they are shorter, and therefore closer to the ground, children are exposed to greater amounts of lead pollution from car exhausts than adults. Their metabolic rate, and the fact that they tend to be in constant physical motion, also makes lead all the more dangerous for them. At least until a certain age, they are more likely to place dirty and dusty objects, including their fingers, into their mouths.

However, when a substance is being tested by a toxicologist, the usual procedure is to choose a group of healthy animals, quite similar to each other in age, who are then fed a similar and nutritious diet. These are then challenged with one single agent.

The results are bound to be quite different when an average cross section of the population, including the young and old people on different diets, is exposed to dozens, even hundreds of substances simultaneously.

The Case of Tartrazine

When a group of rats was exposed to tartrazine (yellow) additives, those who were fed a diet that was perfectly balanced in respect to proteins, carbohydrates, vitamins, and minerals, but was purified, were very badly affected. The yellow additive was, in fact, toxic to them.

When the same additive was given to a group of rats fed on a natural diet, such as they would normally obtain in their environment, the animals showed no ill effects, although that diet may not have been as perfectly balanced as the purified, supplemented one. Apparently the difference was caused by the fact that the first diet did not supply fibers!

ALCOHOL

CHAPTER 11

"Beer makes you feel the way you ought to feel without beer." So said the great Australian writer Henry Lawson. This statement applies to any kind of alcohol, not just beer, because, after all, alcohol is a mood-altering drug.

In moderation, alcohol makes most people feel happy and be lots of fun, and it aids digestion, helps prevent heart disease, and perhaps even helps you live a little longer—that is, if you drink it in moderation.

There is little doubt that we are getting more and more health conscious and that people are beginning to realize that what you put in your mouth has an enormous bearing on your health. However, when it comes to applying this realization to alcohol, we stop short. We are drinking more alcoholic concoctions than ever.

The Metabolism of Alcohol

Alcohol has been with us since time immemorial. A special enzyme with the exclusive task of breaking down alcohol exists in the human liver. This enzyme is called alcohol dehydrogenase, and it probably evolved to enable primitive man to digest fermented fruit fallen to the ground in prehistoric forests.

The effects of alcohol are caused by a mood-altering and toxic substance called ethyl alcohol. It is a clear and volatile substance that is followed by the action of yeast on fruit juices, and there is about one tablespoon of ethyl alcohol in standard beer.

Ethyl alcohol dissolves in both water and fat and reaches practically every organ in the body (including the spinal column, brain cells, and bones) within a few minutes of being ingested. The results of drinking depend not so much on the quantity of alcohol drunk but on the amount of ethyl alcohol that reaches the bloodstream and how quickly it gets there. The faster it gets into the bloodstream, the more potent are its effects.

Roughly 5 percent of what you drink is absorbed directly from the stomach into the bloodstream, and the remainder passes through a living "valve" called the pyloric sphincter before ending up in the small intestine, where it is also absorbed into the bloodstream.

The pylorus is a muscular ring that contracts when the chemical composition of the foodstuffs in the stomach is inappropriate or when there is too much food. If the pylorus can be kept shut, or only slightly open, this will slow down the movement of alcohol. Therefore, alcohol taken on an empty stomach moves through quickly, and its effects are quite powerful—as every drinker knows only too well.

Food delays the absorption of alcohol considerably, irrespective of whether it is eaten before or with the drink. Fatty, oily foods are especially valuable in slowing down the movement of alcohol through the pyloric sphincter.

Sparkling wines, champagne, or spirits with soda contain carbon dioxide and the bubbles "tickle" the pylorus, causing it to open. This is one of the reasons why you can get quite drunk on a relatively weak beverage, such as spumante.

After alcohol reaches the blood it goes to the liver, then to the heart and lungs. It then races through the entire body, eventually getting to the brain, where it stimulates the production of endorphins, which act as an anesthetic.

The only way to get sober is to get the alcohol out of the blood, and you can do this only via urine, breath, sweat, and liver action. Although it may seem like more, only about 3 percent of alcohol leaves via the urine, and around 5 percent leaves via sweat and breath. The rest has to be broken down (oxidized) by the liver. It takes about one hour for the liver to dispose of the alcohol contained in one standard drink. The liver has to be in good condition to do this, and it should not be already overburdened with taking care of other toxins.

HOW THE LIVER DEALS WITH ALCOHOL

The liver is the only organ that does not get its energy from blood sugar; it uses proteins instead. For the liver to function properly it needs a good balance of proteins, vitamins, and minerals.

Often alcoholics have an unbalanced diet that is high in calories but poor in nutrients and proteins, which means that the liver has to work overtime to clear large amounts of alcohol without having the necessary proteins and nutrients for optimal function.

Because alcohol is high in calories, a heavy drinker may satisfy most, if not all, of his or her energy needs without eating a thing. For this and other reasons, it has always been thought that the many health problems associated with alcoholism were, in fact, caused by malnutrition.

Chronic alcohol consumption can cause irritation and inflammation of the linings of the stomach, intestine, and pancreas, severely impairing the absorption of nutrients. It can also impair the liver's ability to handle acetaldehyde, which is the principal product of alcohol and a very toxic substance that can cause damage to the liver.

Acetaldehyde interferes with the activation of vitamins by the liver cells, and the enzyme responsible for breaking down alcohol in the liver, alcohol dehydrogenase, seems to be dependent on vitamin C. This has been described as the metabolic trap suffered by many alcoholics. Many scientists also believe that acetaldehyde is responsible for the effects of alcohol on the heart, the brain, and the dependence caused by the drinking in the first place.

Liver cells get rid of the excess hydrogen formed by alcohol by shunting it into the formation of alphaglycerophosphates and fatty acids. These are the precursors of triglycerides, notoriously implicated in both liver damage and heart and circulatory disorders.

A condition known as hyperlipemia is now established as one of the major predisposing factors in cardiovascular disease, and one that is entirely correctable simply by avoiding alcohol.

Alcohol also competes with other drugs for detoxification so that their metabolism is slowed down and any of their dangerous effects are enhanced. This is why alcohol can kill when mixed with some medications, especially tranquilizers.

IS IT ONLY ALCOHOLICS WHO SUFFER
LIVER DAMAGE FROM ALCOHOL?

Charles Lieber carried out an interesting experiment that he reported in the article "Alcohol and Nutrition" (*Scientific American* 234, no. 3 [1976]: 25). A group of volunteers were fed a good, low-fat diet in which proteins accounted for 25 percent of the calories. They were also given ample vitamin and mineral supplements. They were asked to drink six standard drinks per day for 18 days.

Routine thin-needle biopsy revealed a progressive rise in liver fat after only a few days, and by the end of the 18 days the increase was on the order of eightfold! There were also striking changes (enlargement and distortion) in the mitochondria, while the sites of enzymes associated with the metabolism of alcohol (smooth membranes of the endoplasmic reticulum) proliferated.

It is for this and other reasons that some heavy drinkers show a temporary increase in their capacity to metabolize alcohol so that for a while, perhaps many years, they can drink everybody else "under the table."

These changes occurred following a moderate intake of alcohol by healthy, well-fed people who at no stage showed any symptoms of intoxication. Drunkenness is not necessary to cause liver damage!

Alcohol Addiction

Alcohol is broken down into acetaldehyde. Acetaldehyde may bind to several of the brain's neurotransmitters and form complexes that act as "pseudotransmitters."

One of the reactions of these pseudotransmitters is to form endorphins, the brain's own natural opiates, which explains the ability of alcohol to reduce pain and produce pleasant sensations.

Unfortunately, it also points to one of the reasons why alcohol is so addictive: if acetaldehyde increases the production of opiates in the brain, it is easy to see why one would become addicted to its effects. This is much the same as the way joggers become addicted to endorphins and gamblers to adrenaline.

The Effects of Alcohol

The effects of alcohol are both physiological and psychological. Following are some of the major physiological effects:

PHYSIOLOGICAL EFFECTS

- Alcohol enlarges blood vessels so that you tend to feel warmer. This is only an illusion, however, because alcohol actually enhances heat losses and therefore lowers your resistance to cold weather. Dilated blood vessels can often be seen on the nose and cheeks of heavy drinkers.

- Alcohol affects blood pressure. If you suffer from high blood pressure and drink more than five drinks per day (two drinks per day for women), treating your high blood pressure is a waste of time, as the alcohol pushes the blood pressure up anyway.

- Cardiomyopathy, an irreversible weakening of the heart muscle, can be caused by excess alcohol. However, it has been shown that moderate drinking can dilate coronary arteries and therefore relieve high blood pressure, thus lowering the risk of coronary thrombosis. This paradoxical effect may explain why statistics show that moderate drinkers die of heart attacks less often than those who do not drink at all.

- Alcohol can cause gastritis—chronic inflammation and thickening of the stomach lining. It can also affect the lining of the intestine and the pancreas.

- Alcohol causes various problems in the liver. See the section "How the liver deals with alcohol," page 155.

- Alcohol has been associated with an increased risk of cancer in the upper respiratory and digestive systems. Heavy drinkers often smoke a lot, which compounds the risk of getting cancer.

- Alcohol leads to biochemical abnormalities that have many effects on physiology. Among them are the following:

  1. An increase in lactate, which can cause periods of severe anxiety in susceptible individuals.

  2. A decrease in ketosteroids, which can affect sex hormones and create imbalances between various hormones.

3. A decreased tolerance to galactose (a milk sugar).

4. A decrease in oxidation of amines, which can lead to abnormal ratios of important brain chemicals.

5. An increase in fat deposits.

6. Inhibition of blood-sugar formation via gluconeogenesis, thus diminishing energy reserves for the body and the brain.

7. Changes to the energy production of cells.

8. Elevation of uric acid levels.

9. Decreased protein synthesis, which can slow the repair mechanisms of the body.

10. Protein and fat retention in the liver.

11. Depression of glutathione, an antioxidant component necessary in the removal of free radicals.

12. The stimulation of alcohol metabolism by the liver (smooth endoplasmic reticulum) so that, for a while, one seems to be able to hold his alcohol.

PSYCHOLOGICAL EFFECTS

Alcohol dulls pain and depresses those centers in the brain that are responsible for controlling behavior. It lowers inhibitions so that we no longer feel anxious, guilty, or foolish when we behave in an outlandish fashion. Another common effect of alcohol is to make people depressed. The psychological effects of alcohol are very diverse and depend, to a great extent, on the individual.

Alcoholism and Heredity

We now have good evidence that there is a strong inheritance factor in alcoholism and that an addictive substance is actually produced by the brains of people who drink regularly.

Studies show that when the children of alcoholics are adopted by other families, they are just as likely to become alcoholics as are those reared by their biological parents. In other words, in this case it would seem that nature could turn out to be stronger than nurture.

Alcohol and Nutrition

Is it true that alcohol is good for the digestion? Yes and no. Alcohol tends to inhibit some of the enzymes for the breakdown of food, but if taken in moderation or diluted, it can stimulate the secretion of gastric juices, which help the digestion of proteins. To achieve that effect, however, you do not necessarily have to drink alcohol; just the smell of it or even some fumes will get the digestive juices flowing.

Biochemical changes, which vary from individual to individual, dictate exactly what kind of effect alcohol will have on you. If you are the type who becomes a little anxious after drinking, the easiest way to avoid this happening is to take some calcium on an empty stomach well before you start drinking and then some more while you are drinking.

If you are prone to becoming a little depressed when drinking, take some vitamin C with a little zinc in powder form. These will help to speed up the breakdown of alcohol. Another way to help your body get rid of alcohol a little more quickly is to drink large amounts of fruit sugar (fructose). The best way, of course, is with fruit juices.

Of course, you can take something that will slow down your desire to drink. Vitamin B_3 in the niacin or nicotinic acid form is reported to do this. Please note that vitamin B_3 may cause a severe flushing effect. Although this in itself is not harmful, it may frighten you. Some allergic people can have a severe skin rash following the intake of niacin and, if so, should avoid it. Another nutrient that is said to decrease the craving for alcohol and that helps you to remain sober is the common amino acid glutamic acid.

The controversial supplement vitamin B_{15} (pangamic acid) is said to decrease or even reverse some of the effects of alcohol on the liver. The Russians have been using it for years and swear by it.

THE HANGOVER

If you are only a moderate drinker, a session with a half a dozen drinks may give you a nasty time the morning after. The symptoms of a hangover vary greatly among individuals but can include any of the following: vomiting, loss of appetite, headache, sleeplessness, tiredness, a loss of balance and/or coordination, thirst, and a feeling that your muscles and joints are not up to the job of supporting and propelling you anywhere further than the nearest armchair.

The reasons for all this are the following:

- You have drunk more than your liver has been able to cope with, and the extra alcohol is still circulating in your bloodstream.

- Alcohol blocks the stress signals so that as the brain "wakes up" in the morning it starts to receive all the stress signals at once. It finds it hard to cope with so much so suddenly.

Although some people get headaches from drinking any alcohol, certain wines, especially red ones, seem to affect people more often than others. They contain histamine, which can cause headaches in susceptible people. Some researchers think the tannins (which give wines body and astringent properties) are more likely to be the culprits. Sulfur dioxide, used as an additive and preservative, may also be responsible because it can cause bronchial constriction. It is certainly unhealthy for asthmatics!

More recently, it has been discovered that substances called congeners, which provide most of the taste, smell, and color of different drinks, may be an important factor in alcohol-related headaches. Congeners are made from wood alcohol and fuel oil, both of which are very toxic even in relatively small amounts. They can cause blindness and enlarge the arteries of the brain in much the same way as histamines are said to do. Vodka is a drink that is low in congeners, while whisky, brandy, and red wines have a high content of congeners.

Allergies and Alcohol

If you are allergic to some foods and are on a special diet, remember that alcoholic beverages fall into three categories: spirits, wines, and beers.

Spirits are a fermentation of wheat, barley, or potatoes; wines are made from grapes, which need no added yeast because their skin has a natural yeast; and beers are made of barley and yeast, with or without hops.

Mixing drinks is tantamount to mixing and increasing total congeners (there is always some scientific truth in old wives' tales!). Hence, the hangovers tend to become fiercer as the cocktails become more exotic. So if you are having a great night out and sample a little of that delicate white wine, and some of the gutsy red, plus a little predinner cocktail, with a brandy after dinner, the chances are your hangover will be worse than if you kept to one type of drink. One of the solutions to reducing hangovers is to drink the same beverage and to choose ones that are low in congeners—these usually have less aroma.

THIRST

Thirst is a common result of drinking alcohol. It is not, however, caused by dehydration but by an unhealthy rearrangement of your body fluids. Alcohol causes water to spill out of cells and into the extracellular fluid, thus making you thirsty and causing some extra pressure in your head. This phenomenon will also make your eyes look red and bloodshot in the morning.

SLEEP

Alcohol interferes with rapid eye movement (REM) sleep, which is essential for the recuperating period to have a positive effect. Without a reasonable amount of REM sleep one tends to be tired, irritable, and anxious.

One of the simplest insurances for drinkers is to take a multimineral-multivitamin tablet plus some vitamin B_1 (thiamine) every day. According to Professor Byron Kakulas, head of the Department of Neuropathology at Royal Perth Hospital, a leading neurologist who is a world authority on the effects of alcohol on the brain, "Many of the effects of alcohol can be nullified by taking a few vitamins, especially thiamine which would immediately reduce one of the most common organic mental disorders associated with alcohol."

HOW TO DECREASE THE EFFECTS OF HANGOVERS

- Alcohol is a diuretic, so drink lots of fluids before and after imbibing.
- Drink some fruit juices, as this will help your liver metabolize acetaldehyde a little faster.
- Take some B-complex vitamins, perhaps with a dash of antacid.

- Eat before and while you are drinking, as this slows down the absorption of the alcohol. Milk, fats, and oils line the stomach, while starches absorb some of the alcohol.

- Have some vitamin C, as this not only helps to absorb the alcohol but also helps the liver to break down the alcohol.

- Avoid drinking several different types of alcohol or alcohols that have high amounts of congeners.

- Stay up for a couple of hours after you finish drinking and sleep late.

- According to research in America, oil of evening primrose is said to prevent and cure hangovers.

How to Break the Alcohol Cycle

DRUG THERAPY

Propranolol, a beta blocker used in the treatment of high blood pressure and anxiety, has been suggested as suitable medication for alcoholics. When taken together with alcohol, propranolol seems to block the mood-altering effects of liquor.

As most people drink expecting a change in the way they feel, they may reduce, or stop, their alcohol intake when no such change occurs. It is also possible that the anxiety-reducing effects of the drug may play a role, as many people suspect it is one of the factors that drives people to drink in the first place.

Be that as it may, there seems to be a considerable amount of evidence suggesting that the outcome of treatment of alcoholism is not significantly affected by the form of treatment used. A comprehensive American study, the Rand report (*New Scientist*, December 1983, p. 749), concluded that:

> Perhaps the most important finding . . . is that there are few noteworthy differences among remission rates for various treatment types. Regardless of the setting in which treatment occurs, remissions appear quite uniform, fluctuating by 100 percent at most . . . despite the manifest differences in philosophy, organization and treatment procedures among the sample centers.

However, some forms of treatment not covered by the Rand report demand some attention.

NUTRITIONAL SUPPLEMENTS

NIACIN

Russell Smith is an American physician who has been involved in the treatment of alcoholics in American hospitals since the 1940s. In 1973, and again in 1978, he completed and reported (*Journal of Orthomolecular Psychiatry* 7, no. 1 [1978]: 53) on the results of a five-year study with 500 diagnosed alcoholics who were treated with large doses of vitamin B_3 in the form of nicotinic acid (niacin).

> "Nicotinamide (another form of vitamin B_3) proved of no value to alcoholics, suggesting perhaps another mechanism of action. Nicotinic acid improved sleep patterns, mood stability, and overall functioning in 60 percent of the test group who showed the more serious organic symptoms of the disease. Nicotinic acid significantly reduced acquired tolerance to alcohol and appeared to shorten the course of the acute toxic brain syndrome while all but eliminating the 'dry drunk syndrome': hyperexcitable manic episodes and serious, potentially suicidal depression."

Nicotinic acid crosses the blood-brain barrier easily and tends to inhibit tryptamine while reducing the levels of serotonin and dopamine. Elevated brain levels of these two chemicals have been associated with psychiatric disorders and behavioral abnormalities.

Noradrenaline levels may also be suppressed by nicotinic acid, but, more importantly, Smith suggests that nicotinic acid can stimulate

The Hair of the Dog

Does the hair of the dog help with hangovers? Having a drink the next morning will help a hangover because the methanol enzymes prefer ethanol. So one more drink will shift their attention, so to speak, away from methanol, and less of its nasty by-products will be formed—for a while at least.

histamine and act as a governor of brain catecholamines in general. Histamine itself tends to inhibit monoamine oxidase reactions, a factor that could account for its mood-elevating properties and antidepressant activity. I have used niacin therapy as part of my treatment of alcoholics with considerable success.

HISTAMINE, VITAMINS, MINERALS, & DIETARY MANIPULATIONS

Dr. Oscar Kruesi, of the Huxley Institute for Bio Social Research in New York, has developed another approach to alcoholism that is based on regulating histamine levels with vitamins, minerals, and dietary manipulations.

We have known for some time that histamine may be a neurotransmitter: two of the world's leading experts on brain biochemistry, Snyder and Axelford, claim it is, but we had to wait for Dr. Carl Pfeiffer, of the New Jersey Neuropsychiatric Institute, for confirmation of this fact during the 1970s.

Some of the Benefits of Alcohol

Statistical studies have shown that moderate drinkers tend to live slightly longer than teetotalers, longer than exdrinkers, and longer than people who drink more than three to four drinks per day.

- Drinking with meals seems to help the digestion. Perhaps alcohol stimulates the protein-splitting enzymes. It may also put the drinker in a good mood, something that in itself favors good food assimilation, higher immune resistance, and better blood circulation.

- Blood pressure was found to be lowest among people who drink three or fewer drinks per day. However, it increases progressively with each drink after that and almost doubles at six or more drinks per day.

- The key to minimizing the bad effects of drinking appears to be to drink with meals, and then to drink only in moderation—no more than two to three glasses of wine per day.

There are, in the human body, two separate histamine receptors: H_1 and H_2 H_1 involves well-established allergic responses, and H_2 is a brain histamine receptor (*Nature* 272 [1972]: 329).

Pfeiffer discovered that there are two groups of alcoholics, who have either very high or very low histamine levels. In the treatment of alcoholism it is very important to know to which group the patient belongs. For information about the high and low histamine levels, see page 25.

Alcohol and Its Effect on the Brain

Dr. Jean Lennane, past director of Drug and Alcohol Services at Rozelle and Gladesville Psychiatric Hospital, conducted research into the extent of alcohol-related brain damage in people who regularly consume alcohol.

In 1983 the *Sun Herald* reported that "Australians drink an average of 2.4 drinks per man, woman and child every day of their lives." Dr. Lennane estimates that considering children do not usually drink and that 15 percent of adults are teetotalers, the rest must drink a lot more than 2.4 glasses per day.

Two hundred cases had been assessed up to April 1983, and the youngest case reported was a 34-year-old journalist who, after having four drinks per day for ten years and one final binge, ended up in the hospital with severe frontal lobe damage and impaired memory. The condition of this patient is irreversible.

Alcohol and Osteoporosis

Women who drink large amounts of alcohol are ten times more likely to develop osteoporosis. Calcium supplements will not help if you drink more than one bottle of beer per day, or its equivalent, according to Dr. Richard Evans of the Metabolic Unit of the Concord Hospital in Sydney.

Dr. Lennane is careful with her pronouncements: "Not every social drinker will suffer brain damage. Some people are more tolerant than others. The danger is we don't know yet who is at risk." Often, it is not the alcoholic or the derelict on skid row who we should worry about but the ordinary person who steadily consumes alcohol every day.

Dr. Lennane suggests that anyone who has eight or more drinks per day should have an assessment of his or her ability to function normally.

LOSS OF ADAPTABILITY

The frontal lobes of the brain are often affected by alcohol. At worst, people affected by alcohol have a great deal of difficulty in organizing simple tasks or lack the incentive to do anything. At best, their organizing skills, which depend on frontal lobes, are diminished.

Frontal lobe damage is insidious because people still retain their normal intelligence but lose the ability to work out whether they have a problem or not—let alone do something about it. Many people do not realize this until they are presented with a new set of problems that demand the ability to adjust.

The habitual drinker loses his capacity to adapt. As little as a couple of drinks per day over some years can cause chronic impairment of intelligence. Drinking can cause the brain to actually shrink because of cell death. This results in memory loss, decreased intelligence, impairment of thinking, and alterations to personality.

Alcohol the Drug

Alcohol is a drug in every sense of the word. It is, in fact, a mood-altering drug with profound short-term and long-term effects on almost every part of the human body and most facets of human physiology, particularly on the biochemistry of the brain. If alcohol were discovered today and a pharmaceutical company tried to market it, I doubt that it would be allowed without a doctor's prescription!

IMPAIRED INTELLIGENCE

One feature of intelligence that may suffer as a result of chronic alcohol consumption, perhaps even at moderate or "social drinking" levels, is crystallized intelligence. This is defined as the ability to use an accumulated body of general information to make judgments and solve problems.

In practical terms, crystallized intelligence is that used in understanding the various facets of an argument, understanding the real meaning of newspaper editorials, or dealing with problems for which there are no clear answers but only better or worse options. By the time one arrives at that stage, however, it is often too late for total recovery.

THE CHEMISTRY OF LOVE

There is sex and there is love, and there are love without sex and sex without love as well as sexual love. Everybody knows what being colorblind means, and it may surprise you that there is a disease that causes some people to become "love blind."

Such people are normal in every respect: they may be very friendly, sociable individuals who often form close relationships with members of the opposite sex and may even get married, but they cannot experience the intense feeling of passion known as "being in love" any more than a colorblind person can discern the brilliant shades and hues of a colorful painting.

As humanity moves away from its poetic and religious past toward the robotic future of the 21st century, we are discovering that love blindness is only one of the many psychosexual problems that stem, at least in part, from neuroendocrinological fluctuations and imbalances. Loss of libido, separation anxiety, hysteroid dysphoria, delusional love, dependence syndrome, paranoid jealousy, hypomanic love, and obsessive infatuation are some of the new labels believed to be closely linked with the deranged brain chemistry of some interpersonal relationships.

Being in love is one of the most intense personal experiences possible, and, like most of our moods, there are some chemical changes within our brains that are associated with it. Anyone who has ever been in love knows that it is a state somewhat reminiscent of madness, hyperactivity, and hallucination.

According to Dr. Michael Liebowitz, a neurophysiologist at Columbia University in New York, there are three basic types of love:

1. There is the adrenaline kind, which is characterized by the orgasmic, hedonistic pursuit of sexual arousal and fulfillment.

2. There is romantic love, in which the brain manufactures large quantities of a group of chemicals called enkephalines, which can lessen the sensation of pain but may also be responsible for hallucinations, delusions, and a remarkable inability to think clearly.

3. There is marital love, which is thought to be associated with an increased production of natural opiates (a group of morphine–like substances that dull the senses) in the brain.

THE BRAIN'S NATURAL OPIATES

When you are in love, you feel "high," and some people may have noticed the similarity between the withdrawal symptoms associated with the breakup of relationships and those elicited by amphetamine withdrawal.

One of the reasons for this is that an "in love" brain manufactures more phenylethylalanine, a chemical derived from phenylalanine, an amino acid found in many foods. As soon as an affair starts to turn sour, the brain halts, or drastically reduces, its output of phenylethylalanine, and the person involved begins to suffer withdrawal symptoms.

Dr. Donald Kline and Dr. Michael Liebowitz conducted an in-depth study of such people and found that a considerable number of them tended to go on a chocolate binge as soon as they began to suffer some of the depression associated with the breakup of their relationship. Why chocolate? Because this gastronomic delight is extracted from the seeds of *Theobroma cacao* (which literally means "food of the gods"), and its main constituent, theobromine, is a stimulant. Chocolate is also rich in phenylalanine.

Phenylalanine is also used by the brain to make norepinephrine (noradrenaline) and to slow down the breakdown of natural opiates (the endorphins and enkephalines), which are responsible for, among other things, lowering the sensation of pain. An increased intake of phenyl-alanine may result in higher brain levels of endorphins and therefore a decreased sensitivity to pain. So it stands to reason that phenylalanine could be useful as a sort of natural painkiller or antidepressant.

The pain of being in love, if the love is not reciprocated or the affair is terminated, can be as debilitating as any psychiatric illness, and it may well be that phenylalanine, or chocolate, could be used by lovers to reduce the intensity of their lovesickness.

HORMONE STIMULATION

The hypothalamus is in charge of our behavior in general and our sexual tendencies in particular. This small portion of the brain, which is also known as a neuroendocrinal transducer, translates inputs (transduces) from our external and internal environments into special chemicals known as releasing factors, which are a type of hormone. These in turn travel to the pituitary gland and cause it to release its various hormones, which are then circulated to reach the various endocrine glands, which, thus stimulated, begin to pour out their hormones.

In simple terms, when a man looks into the eyes of the woman he loves, what he sees is first changed from light impulses to electrical

Foods Containing Phenylalanine

almonds	egg
apple	herring
avocado	milk
baked beans	parsley
beef	peanuts
beet	pineapple
carrot	soybeans
chicken	soy proteins
chocolate	spinach
cottage cheese	tomato

pulsations. These move along the optic nerves and reach the brain, where they are again transformed by the hypothalamus into releasing factors, which eventually cause adrenal hormones to make his heart beat faster. This can also happen with olfactory stimulation by the subtle, often barely discernible pheromones. Though the influence of scents on sexual behavior is not recognized at a conscious level, other stimulants can produce dramatic effects, and it may well be that people with blockages along one of these circuits turn out to be love blind.

People suffering with decreased pituitary function (hypopituitarism) often have problems with their feelings. However, in sexual matters, it is the hypothalamus that sends luteinizing hormone releasing factors (LHRF) to the pituitary, which then pours out two separate hormones, follicle stimulating hormone (FSH) and luteinizing hormone (LH). FSH instructs the testes to start sperm production, and LH is responsible for the production of testosterone—the male sex hormone.

While it might seem that the hypothalamus is responsible for fueling sexual encounters, perhaps it is the brain's own opiates (phenylalanine) that may be responsible for keeping couples together.

People may cling desperately to their partners to keep up their production of phenylethylalanine and therefore avoid withdrawal. Perhaps they are unwittingly using their partners as mood regulators!

However, like anything, too much of a good thing can be harmful, and excessive amounts of the brain's own opiates can cause people to become insensitive or dulled to physical and emotional interaction.

Aphrodisiacs

Mankind's search for aphrodisiacs has driven people to swathe themselves in colorful clothes and exotic scents. They have eaten anything that even remotely resembles a sex organ (bananas, oysters, and rhinoceros horn) as well as the actual sex organs of animals.

Luteinizing hormone releasing factor (LHRF) has recently been dubbed "the ultimate aphrodisiac" following reports that it has effects that are highly specific to sexual behavior. Robert Moss, professor of physiology at the University of Texas Health Science Center in Dallas, reports that it seems to improve the sexual functioning of some impotent males.

LHRF is also being tested as a contraceptive for both males and females, and it has been found that while LHRF enhances female libido, there may be some cases where the opposite is true for males.

Dopamine, a neurotransmitter partially involved in sex, is made from tyrosine, a common amino acid now available as a food supplement. However, too much dopamine can be responsible for certain mental illnesses.

Serotonin, made from tryptophan, excites but can depress the male sex drive. Eggs, lecithin, and choline, helped along by vitamin B_1, can aid in the synthesis of acetylcholine, and researchers at Tulane University in New Orleans claim acetylcholine can have dramatic effects on human sexual behavior.

Meanwhile, would-be Romeos may try the local fruit shop. While various perfume makers have been desperately trying to find a sex-

Chocolate Addiction

So pleasant is the stimulation from chocolate that some people use it almost as a drug. During the 16th century the Spanish government, under pressure from the church, which disapproved of anyone being "stimulated," banned chocolate because it claimed that it was a "drink of the devil"!

Like prohibitions on all mood-altering substances ever discovered, the only effect this had was to spread the use of chocolate further and make it more desirable and expensive.

In the ancient markets of Mexico chocolate was actually used as currency. The courtesans of Louis XV used it as a sexual stimulant, and *Cosmopolitan* magazine voted it among the top ten aphrodisiacs.

In a sense, however, chocolate may be considered a drug, and, like all drugs, it can cause addiction if taken too often. This, of course, gives rise to the depression of withdrawal when chocolate is not available.

attractant scent, a spray-on aphrodisiac, researchers have been looking at androsterone, a potent male hormone that is said to attract females.

The lowly vegetable celery apparently contains some androsterone, which is released through perspiration after digestion. I am told that people find it irresistible, although it is not detected consciously and I am not sure whether your partner will want to cuddle or nibble you after a celery binge, but it may well be a healthier and sexier alternative to expensive perfume!

INDEX

OTHER ULYSSES PRESS HEALTH BOOKS:

COUNT OUT CHOLESTEROL

Art Ulene, M.D. and Val Ulene, M.D.

Complete with counter and detailed dietary plan, this companion resource to the *Count Out Cholesterol Cookbook* shows how to design a cholesterol-lowering program that's right for you. $12.95

COUNT OUT CHOLESTEROL COOKBOOK

Art Ulene, M.D. and Val Ulene, M.D.

A companion guide to *Count Out Cholesterol*, this book shows you how to bring your cholesterol levels down with the help of 250 gourmet recipes. $14.95

HOW TO CUT YOUR MEDICAL BILLS

Art Ulene, M.D. and Val Ulene, M.D.

This handy book offers insiders tips known only to health professionals and savvy patients. It shows how to save money on doctor bills, hospital costs, drug prescriptions, and much more. $11.95

THE VITAMIN STRATEGY

Art Ulene, M.D. and Val Ulene, M.D.

A game plan for good health, this book helps readers design a vitamin and mineral program tailored to their individual needs. $11.95

DISCOVERY PLAY

Art Ulene, M.D. and Steven Shelov, M.D.

This book guides parents through the first three years of their child's life, offering play activity with a special emphasis on nurturing self-esteem. $9.95

TAKE IT OFF! KEEP IT OFF!

Art Ulene, M.D.

> This best-selling weight-loss book offers a 28-day program for taking off the pounds and keeping them off forever. $9.95

LAST WISHES: A HANDBOOK TO GUIDE YOUR SURVIVORS

Lucinda Page Knox, M.S.W. and Michael D. Knox, Ph.D.

> This simple do-it-yourself workbook helps people put their affairs in order and eases the burden on their survivors. *Last Wishes* allows readers to plan their own funeral, design a memorial, and leave final instructions and messages for their survivors. $12.95

IRRITABLE BOWEL SYNDROME: A NATURAL APPROACH

Rosemary Nicol

> This book offers a natural approach to a problem millions of sufferers have. The author clearly defines the symptoms and diagnosis, and then offers a dietary and stress-reduction program for relieving the effects of this disease. $9.95

KNOW YOUR BODY: THE ATLAS OF ANATOMY

Introduction by Trevor Weston, M.D.

> Designed to provide a comprehensive and concise guide to the structure of the human body, this book offers more than 250 color illustrations. An easy-to-follow road map of the human body. $11.95

To order these or other Ulysses Press books call 800-377-2542 or write to Ulysses Press, P.O. Box 3440, Berkeley, CA 94703-3440. All retail orders are shipped free of charge. California residents must include sales tax. Allow two to three weeks for delivery.

About the Author

William Vayda, one of Australia's pioneers in orthomolecular medicine and psychiatry, specializes in nutritional and environmental medicine. He is particularly involved in the treatment of chronic fatigue, postviral syndromes, and disorders of immunity, especially allergic syndromes (asthma, candida, arthritis), and psychiatric disorders related to nutritional problems.

A graduate osteopath, William Vayda first became interested in the role of nutrition in psychiatry and obtained postgraduate diplomas in nutrition–naturopathy, acupuncture, and clinical hypnotherapy.

Vayda was appointed senior lecturer in physiology and nutrition at the Sydney College of Chiropractic and Osteopathy in 1973 and later taught differential diagnosis and clinical nutrition. The following year he founded the Australian Institute for Orthomolecular Research.

In the late 1970s, Vayda ran a training program for medical doctors and other health professionals and ran special postgraduate courses in nutritional and environmental medicine and psychiatry.

Working as a clinician and diagnostician with a group of open-minded and progressive medical scientists, Vayda carried out extensive research into the role of nutrition in mental illness and the role of allergies and chemicals in asthma and immunological disorders.

William Vayda is president of the International College of Applied Nutrition (Australia) and a fellow of the Oceania College of Clinical Nutrition. He is a member of the International Association of Orthomolecular Medicine, the Australasian Society of Orthomolecular Psychiatry, the Huxley Institute for Bio-Social Research, the New York Academy of Science, and the Australian Natural Therapists Association (ANTA).

Vayda has lectured extensively at universities, medical schools, and various naturopathic colleges and to the general public. He is a well-known and prolific writer of popular columns and scientific papers. He is a contributing editor of *Wellbeing* magazine and has written several best-selling books, including *Health for Life: Are You Allergic to the 20th Century?*, *The Candida Questions and Answers Book*, and *Chronic Fatigue, the Silent Epidemic*.